MYSTICAL MOTHERHOOD

Create a Happy and Conscious Family:

A Guidebook for Conception,

Pregnancy, Birth and Beyond

Pritam Atma, FNP

DEDICATED TO THE DIVINE MOTHER

"I am working to bring peace to the earth, all we need is one kid

and one womb and one woman and one man."

—YOGI BHAJAN

April 8, 1982

TABLE OF CONTENTS

INTRODUCTION

This is an experiment. It is a revolution. We are creating a new model of the family unit by demonstrating a different path to raise conscious children and awaken the true potential within individuals. It is time to stop repeating the same patterns that have been passed down one generation after another and raise children who are reality centered, focused, spontaneous, respectful, humorous, ethical, open-minded, creative, and deeply connected. This book is a call to action and was written specifically for mothers. If the frequency of women changes, as they are the ones who birth new life into this world, so will the entire human race. We are on the verge of an awakening, and you are the change makers. It takes grace and grit to challenge status quo.

There is a deep sense of insecurity and pressure in the world, and people are desperately looking for something that will help to relieve their feelings of unease. Mothers, in particular, are suffering from isolation and depression at higher rates than ever before and are in need of guidance. The transition into parenthood is a unique time when adults are open to change and ready to improve for the sake of their children. I am providing parents with the opportunity to invest in the growth and development of their children by teaching them to model healthy behavior so that their family can find happiness.

This book provides a roadmap to awakening and healthy living using Abraham Maslow's hierarchy of needs as a guidepost to help you meet the physiological, safety, love, and esteem needs in order to become a fulfilled family. Within these pages there are forty alternative, yet practical, concepts surrounding motherhood and wellbeing that combine Eastern and Western philosophy from some of the world's leading provocative thinkers. You will find new insights on nutrition, creativity, Kundalini Yoga and Meditation, self-development, and holistic health. You will also find exercises or meditations at the end of many sections, which will help guide you into living your highest self. The hierarchy of needs is an ongoing process of growth and many of the needs are intertwined. It is unique as individuals can approach it in a chronological order or enter at a stagnant stage of growth. This guidebook can be read in a similar manner.

Maslow's theory provides a platform to completely transform and awaken both the parents and children within families. The hierarchy enables people to work up from satisfying their most basic needs to completing their greatest achievements, and it is applicable to each member of the family no matter what stage they are at. Readers will learn to create physical, emotional, and spiritual balance through the transitions of conception, pregnancy, birth, postpartum, childhood, and adulthood. You will learn how to raise conscious and creative children, and you will also gain a better understanding of how to improve your personal health, wellbeing, and spiritual connection. This book was created to help you reach a higher state of consciousness, which is really a deeper connection to yourself and ultimately to the wellbeing of the entire human race. You will begin to question the way things have always been done and experience a new way of Being that may cause you to feel better. We are not bending to society's norms or listening to authority but ingraining a new way to raise children by altering the habits of adults. Here are the basics of the hierarchy of needs adjusted to fit the needs of mothers and their children.

1. Physiological needs help to maintain a healthy body and mind, and we must have our basic needs met in order to create a strong foundation for our lives. Here you will find an alternative outlook on nutrition, fertility, reducing toxic load, enhancing the home environment, and

changing your sleep patterns to connect to higher states of wellbeing. This section will help families to consciously prepare for a child or improve their already busy household.

2. Safety needs begin in the womb, and children do not grow or achieve unless they feel protected. Here I provide a plan for a conscious pregnancy, safe birth, and a healing postpartum period, which is vital for mothers and newborns. In this section, you will prepare for your birth, learn how to heal yourself, and take care of your baby.

3. Love and belonging needs are a part of our tribal nature. We need to feel loved and accepted by our parents and in our relationships. In this section, I guide readers to take a more conscious approach to how they raise their children by providing a new outlook for the relationship they have within themselves and others. Mothers will learn how to care for themselves during pregnancy, postpartum, and beyond.

4. Esteem needs help us to create higher positions in a group and feel respected. Here we examine concepts such as achievement, mastery, independence, status, self-respect, and respect from others. Parents will learn how to approach their child in the early childhood years through conscious development, bonding, and enhanced growth.

5. Self-actualization, self-fulfillment, being fully human, or living a no-limits life occurs when we realize our true potential and take the path of our ultimate destiny. I will discuss the qualities of a self-actualized individual such as honesty, intrinsic motivation, and connection to the larger universe. Parents will learn how to ultimately cultivate creativity, advanced expression, and appreciation within themselves and their children.

Anxiety, fear, guilt, insecurities, and disappointment do not have to be part of any family experience. You will learn that if you can let go of your mind and ingrained belief systems—and truly trust in your instincts—you can experience the full range of heightened emotion surrounding motherhood including exhaustion, frustration, love, and even euphoria—and learn from them. These emotions are great teachers. Throughout the book, you will find personal birth stories from mothers in their own words. Each anecdote was reproduced as written to maintain authenticity. The handing down of stories provides a unique way of teaching and helps women prepare for birth, reflect on motherhood, and learn from one another. At their core, all women carry an ageless knowing of the divine feminine, and sharing this knowing creates a unified connection. The intensity and harmony that accompanies parenting is a place where families can change and a new generation can rise to their destiny to change the world. I invite you now to take the road to changing yourself and creating conscious families.

ABOUT THE AUTHOR

Pritam Atma (previously named Chelsea Wiley) wrote Mystical Motherhood as part of a series of books on conscious conception and pregnancy. Her second book, *Fertile: Prepare Your Body, Mind, and Spirit for Conception and Pregnancy to Create a Conscious Child,* is also a wonderful resource for women on the path of awakening. Pritam is deeply connected to bringing conscious children into this world. She currently works as a Nurse Practitioner in a fertility center within the New York area practicing Reproductive Medicine. Pritam also works with women privately and in groups, helping them to apply the concepts of the Mystical Motherhood book series to increase their fertility and consciously prepare for motherhood. You can learn more about this at:

www.mysticalmotherhood.com

Facebook: Mystical Motherhood

Instagram: @mysticalmotherhood

iTunes: Mystical Motherhood Podcast

Pritam has also worked as a labor and delivery nurse at the top medical center: the University of California, San Francisco, and studied with Ina May Gaskin, the most famous midwife in the world. She is a board-certified Family Nurse Practitioner (FNP) and a Kundalini Yoga and Meditation teacher. At the hospital and in the primary care clinic, she found that families were unprepared for birth and parenting, that they lacked knowledge to maintain health, and yearned for a deeper understanding of how to integrate spiritual practices into daily life. Pritam envisions raising the consciousness of families across the globe and changing the frequency of the women who bring children into this world so that the next generation can live as peaceful, vibrant, and healthy individuals. She wrote this book for mothers, as she is a mother herself and knows that this population will change the world as we know it.

ABOUT THE ARTIST

Kate Wolfgang Savage is a classically trained fine artist, illustrator and creative consultant. She possesses the unique ability to translate ideas into a cohesive visual language and the skill to express the essential level of artistry. Her artistic expertise lies in substantiating modern ideas with aesthetic tradition and has a special eye and discernment for the ubiquitous humanist themes of classical mythology, persona archetypes and great traditional narratives. Kate's work is most significantly influenced by, but not limited to, the great 19th century naturalists, classical antiquity and vintage art nouveau and art deco.

SECTION I

MEETING YOUR PHYSIOLOGICAL NEEDS BEFORE CONCEPTION

"Undoubtedly these physiological needs are the most prepotent of all needs. What this means specifically is that in the human being who is missing everything in life in an extreme fashion, it is most likely that the major motivation would be the physiological needs rather than any others. A person who is lacking food, safety, love and esteem would most likely hunger for food more strongly than for anything else. If all the needs are unsatisfied and the organism is dominated by the physiological needs, all other needs may become simply nonexistent or be pushed into the background."

– ABRAHAM MASLOW

1. THE CONNECTION BETWEEN YOUR BRAIN AND FOOD

"As your whole system comes into balance, your food will stop poisoning you, your body will begin to repair and heal naturally, your relationships will cease to be emotional battlegrounds, and your sense of separation from nature and Spirit will dissolve."

–ALBERT VILLOLDO

For years I was hellbent on completing the highest degree in my field. At that time in my life, outward accomplishment gave me my sense of self-worth. It was a long and difficult road to become a family nurse practitioner (FNP). I worked forty hours a week while receiving my prerequisites, entered a full-time year-round program for my masters and finished my FNP degree while birthing and raising my two daughters. This is all while moving and watching my husband build a company. We didn't necessarily plan it this way—life just happens—and sometimes we allow it to get too overwhelming. It was not until after I graduated that I realized the full extent of the disease-oriented health-care system the West runs.

I had been living in the realm of hungry ghosts, always looking for the next best thing or accomplishment for fulfillment. Becoming an FNP didn't make me feel happy because it was clear that I wasn't going to be able to help people heal. It is only when we focus on the whole system, the mind, body, and spirit, that people make rapid and lasting changes in their lives. In the clinics, I witnessed a focus on keeping people sick through a cocktail of drugs. The Western medical system ignores the body's natural ability to heal itself and the motivation it takes to get there. There are thousands of medications that address the immediate symptoms, but none can handle the underlying problems that lead to disease. We are very good at attacking diseases and symptoms, but we very rarely get to the root cause.

Doctors tend to be experts in their specific field, but very few ask their patients what foods they are consuming. They like to specialize, and then super specialize, which misses the whole picture of health. I personally witnessed most medical professionals tiptoeing around the massive obesity epidemic that is now America. There are too many emotions, stories, and excuses connected to food, and asking about diet would have opened a can of worms that was too much for them to handle in their limited time slot of twenty minutes per patient. Research is now linking the connection to health and wellbeing to the health of the gut. Childhood obesity is rising and it's time to question the amount of sugar and unprocessed foods that we feed our children and ourselves. This epidemic is also now spreading to other countries around the world. Women need to prepare their bodies for a healthy pregnancy and rid themselves of the high amount of toxins in food and the environment in order to birth healthy children. If we want to change our frequency, reach higher states of consciousness, and birth healthy children, we must detoxify our systems and change our diet.

Simply by avoiding certain foods, you can become more productive, agile during activity, overcome your obstacles, and get a sense of courage to move forward in life. The way we eat has changed more over the last fifty years compared to the last five thousand years. We are eating in a way that is far different than our ancestors did, and we are getting sick. It's time to eliminate the foods that are reducing your energy and making your body sick such as high fructose corn syrup, genetically modified wheat, and hormone-injected dairy. When we know what to avoid eating, our lives begin to change.

In order for us to build a new earth, we need to upgrade our hormones, nervous system, and brain chemistry. Alberto Villoldo, author of *One Spirit Medicine*, wrote an excellent book that creates a connection between our diet, our brain and gut health, and our ability to connect to Spirit and our higher self. He explained that most of the population is running on the limbic brain, which was created for survival and meeting just our basic needs. This part of our brain functions like an animal and is focused on feeding, fighting, fleeing, and fornicating. The human body was not created to operate for just these lower needs, and we are cutting ourselves short of our mind-blowing capabilities when we draw our energy from these lower functions.

The limbic system is the part of the brain that craves sugar and can't turn down comfort foods. It is the center that is obsessed with food, in need of constant sex or attention, and suffers from addiction to mind-dulling drugs and alcohol. When you are emotionally withdrawing, feeling biased or negative toward another person, or filled with destructive behavior, you are functioning from this part of your brain. Most of us are not even aware that we are operating with these types of belief systems, and thus the world is being filled with fear, a lot of guns, and a tendency to run from ourselves. You can see the drive of the limbic system clearly displayed on social media with newsfeeds filled with, fear, food, or sex.

If this is resonating with you or you know someone like this, I have some great news. There is nothing wrong with you! There is just something awry with the neural connections of your brain and your hormonal chemistry, and this can be fixed. We are entering a new age on the planet, and in order for us to be filled with inspiration, creativity, and beauty, we need to start to work from primarily our neocortex and not from the limbic system, which is the mammalian center. We cannot begin to even envision a new future by repeating the past.

The neocortex is the part of our brain that creates music like Mozart and art like Frida Khalo. If you want to leave a legacy or function on a higher level, it is necessary to build new neural pathways in this part of your brain. The neocortex is involved in higher functions such as sensory perception, generation of motor commands, spatial reasoning, conscious thought, and language. If we don't change our neural pathways, we will pass our belief systems down generation after generation, and this planet will remain in destruction. Villoldo discussed the connections between our neural pathway, everyday actions, and our families very well when he said,

"This map contains sights, sounds, scents, memories, and early childhood experiences. It is thought that as many as half of our maps of reality are formed in the womb, as the mother's stress hormones pass through the placental barrier to the fetus. So if your mother was not sure she could count on your father to be there and support her, your map will code for a reality in which you can't count on men to be there for you, or a universe where men will not support your endeavors. If, on the other hand, your mother was confident she could count on her beloved, your mental map will show a world you can count on—and it will create this reality around you."

Creating a healthy brain map is vital when you are getting ready to conceive or are pregnant, especially if you are ready to stop family patterns. As parents, if you want to change the future, you have to change your neural pathways. This can be done through many forms, such as meditation, but also simply by altering your diet to be filled with more plant-based proteins and fats and less sugar and carbohydrates. Next, I am going to discuss ways to rewire your brain for joy.

2. REDUCING YOUR TOXIC LOAD

"Please keep in mind the distinction between healing and treatment: treatment originates from outside, whereas healing comes from within."

—DR. ANDREW WEIL

Albert Villoldo is a shamanic healer who lived in the Amazon for twenty-five years. Villoldo went to the Amazon looking for a cure for cancer and found that none of the tribes in the region had any sickness. Their health span equaled their life span. Their diet held the key to keeping connected directly to Spirit and the secret to joy and serenity. When Albert himself was told that he would die, because the parasites he had contracted through his travels were eating his organs, he began a deep journey of detoxification and provided a road map for changing the body by healing the gut.

The toxic overload humans are facing today makes it much harder to connect to the subtle state of oneness that our ancestors once had, and we must now work much harder to detoxify and repair our bodies. This is especially important if we are carrying children or if you are planning on becoming pregnant. Individuals like Villoldo, many other professionals on the planet, and myself are urging people to clean their diet by eliminating some of the toxins that are damaging the gut and taking away the good bacteria needed for health. There is a great movement toward a diet that lacks gluten and is free of sugar, dairy, genetically modified organisms (GMOs), and heavy metals. It is important to release these toxins but also vital to replenish our system with the nutrients and supplements required to create healthy gut flora.

BREAKING DOWN THE CULPRITS

Grains and Sugar

Grains are toxic for most of us because we have not evolved to function on the grain-based diet of our present time. Albert Villoldo explained that our ancestors ate a plant-based diet high in fat. He explained that we lost the connection between Spirit and the natural world during the agricultural revolution, which was ten thousand years ago. Villoldo said, "During this time we switched from a fat-and-protein-rich Paleolithic hunter-gatherer diet...to a diet based on wheat, barley, rice, and maize—grains with a high glycemic index, or blood-glucose potential." When our ancestors began to live on this high glycemic diet of sugar, the centuries that followed were filled with war and conflict.

To make it even worse, we are not presently eating the same wheat that people were given just seventy-five years ago. To eliminate famine post–World War II, a dwarf wheat was introduced, creating twenty times more gluten in breads than older strains. Gluten is found in most grains including wheat, rye. and barley. The carbohydrates from grain break down into glucose. When we are fueled by sugar rather than a fat-based diet, our moods, stability, and mental functioning are negatively affected.

Villoldo explained that the typical American adult consumes one hundred and fifty pounds of added sugar yearly including fake sugars and those in the forms of processed foods. Imagine what we are teaching our children and how we are affecting their moods. Sugar is constantly being used as a reward for our youth and is also a form of emotional relief. It is one molecule off from heroine and stimulates the same receptors in the brain. Sugar is also one of the greatest addictions on the planet and the leading culprit of bad bacteria in the gut and a sluggish brain.

I personally witnessed an epidemic of childhood obesity in healthcare clinics based out of California, which is supposedly one of the healthier states in the country. I helped to manage eleven- to fourteen-year-old girls and boys diagnosed with high blood pressure and high cholesterol. These patients were taking a lot of medications for their age to control what should have been changed through diet and exercise. One patient, whom we will call Sam, was in a really bad situation and unhealthy state. Not only was he diagnosed with the above at the age of thirteen, but he was also clinically depressed and could not lose the extra one hundred pounds he held because his family kept feeding him the same types of foods. Despite education, they could not see the connection between processed foods and weight gain. They equated "fat free" to "healthy," when these products are higher in sugar, which can be seen by reading the label.

The only way that we are going to change our families, and the future, is to stop passing down these habitual patterns to our innocent children who don't know any better. Many families in the clinics were not as bad as the above example because they chose to make changes slowly and noticed which products their children were physically or emotionally reacting to. There are many dietary changes recommended in this book that need to occur for massive changes in our hearts and minds, but you can take this process slowly if needed. Rome was not built overnight. Pick what feels right for you and for your body, and stick to that; the first step in change is just committing to it.

The Truth About GMOs, Toxins and Heavy Metals

GMOs are crops that make up more than seventy percent of the foods in American stores. The DNA of these crops has been altered to create new and stronger strands so that the products last longer and are resistant to pests in the field. Villoldo explained that ninety percent of the corn grown in the U.S. has been genetically modified by splicing in Bacillus thuringiensis (Bt) bacteria. The industry says that this does not pose a threat to us, yet studies have shown that Bt causes allergic reactions and intestinal damage to rats and farm workers who have been exposed.

Many supporters of GMOs have said that the crops would reduce chemical fertilizers, increase yield, and be used to feed the world's hungry. So far this has not been the case, and many European countries have completely banned the products as they are yet to be proven safe. Independent scientists claim that they can cause food allergies, antibiotic resistance, immune suppression, and toxic reactions. The only way to know that you are not eating a GMO food is by buying foods that are "Certified organic by the USDA."

Roundup is another product to be aware of that is used on crops. It is a pesticide that is believed to alter the DNA of the friendly bacteria in your gut for long periods of time, even after you have stopped eating it. It is commonly found on soy and corn products around America. However, many organic farmers have reported that Roundup was found on their crops despite not using the spray. This is because Monsanto, the company who uses this pesticide, is not properly regulated in the U.S., similar to the case of GMOs. It is important to encourage senators to mandate that independent scientific research studies be conducted on these issues in order not to remain victim to this type of massive food control.

Heavy metals are responsible for more ailments facing our bodies and our planet. Over a very short span we have released thousands of synthesized molecules including flame retardants, nonstick pans, plastic, and medicine in drugs. There is no data on the long-term effects of what these products can do to our health. Villoldo explained that there are eighty-two thousand chemicals approved in the U.S., and only a quarter of them have been tested. Most of these chemicals remain in the environment and affect our food. He said, "Because of the toxins in our brain and nervous system from pesticides and mercury, we can no longer readily experience unity with all creation. No matter how arduously we meditate…" The human brain is not designed to take on this type of toxic overload, and we need to be aware of what we eat, wear, and give to our children.

Dairy

Many conventional milk products such as cheese, yogurt, ice cream, and butter have been altered with a synthetic GE bovine growth hormone (rBGH). Some studies have linked rBGH to elevated risks of cancer. When cows are given this hormone, they have been known to suffer from shortened life spans, mastitis, increased birth defects, and high rates of diseases, infertility, and stress. Antibiotics fed to livestock can enter the human food chain, affecting the way hormones are metabolized in our bodies

Dr. Christiane Northrup, author of *Women's Bodies Women's Wisdom*, explained that women get relief from heavy menstrual bleeding and endometriosis when they stop consuming dairy foods. She saw in her personal practice a link to dairy and chronic vaginal discharge, acne, menstrual cramps, fibroids, and intestinal upset. She noted that the patients who changed to organic dairy products sometimes saw a decrease in these symptoms.

Be willing to attempt to eliminate dairy in your own household for a couple of weeks to see the effect it has on your family. Many parents are worried about reducing calcium intake for their children, which is a normal concern. However, milk is not the best source of calcium, and there are a lot of alternatives including increasing the amount of dark green leafy vegetables such as kale, collards, and broccoli. Our pediatricians were against any dairy after the age of two as they saw more harm in their clinic than benefits. For families whose children suffered from dairy allergies, they encouraged parents to give children organic goat's milk alternating with almond milk and lots of calcium through their food. We personally had one daughter who suffered from a dairy allergy that covered her whole body in eczema or a red rash. She adjusted well to a mix of almond and goat's milk and loves her dark leafy greens, because that is what she has always been offered.

I encourage you to absorb what you can about reducing the toxic overload in your body. Everything does not have to be given up at once. Small changes go a long way. Choose the alterations to your diet that work for your family and go for it. Even buying organic or reading the labels can make vast alterations to health. If you are planning on having a baby, or already have children, reducing the toxic overload through watching what you consume will help to create a better brain and gut connection and ultimately more health and happiness.

3. A SENSIBLE PLAN TO ALTER YOUR DIET

"Don't eat anything your great-great grandmother wouldn't recognize as food. There are a great many food-like items in the supermarket your ancestors wouldn't recognize as food...stay away from these."

–MICHAEL POLLAN

Alejandro Junger, M.D., is another leading expert on the connection between a healthy gut and wellbeing. He has made it his life mission to help people get clean through a healthy diet and has assisted thousands across the world to heal their second brain, the gut. He explained in his book, *Clean Gut*, that there is a connection between poor gut bacteria and depression, allergies, autoimmune diseases, constipation, back pain, infertility, cancer, and heart disease. He described the gut as our GPS system. When not functioning properly, this three-thousand-square-foot tube can cause us to make the wrong decisions in our life and pass this pattern down to our children. When your gut is healthy, you can navigate life properly with a newfound joy and energy. Every single muscle and cell in the body will act properly through nutrition, and it is vital to feed your family right.

You cannot live a long and healthy life, deeply connected to Spirit, or function at your highest limits, if you have an unhealthy gut. By changing your diet, you can ultimately switch from the limbic brain, which feeds on sugar, to the higher brain or the neocortex. By altering your habits, you will also set an example for your children and prepare your bodies for pregnancy through a healthy diet. As a society, if we begin to live like our ancestors did, on a diet rich in plant-based protein and healthy fats with minimal toxins, we will be able to function at our highest level. There is a strong connection between the energetic field of the child a woman births and her overall wellbeing between the time of conception and childbirth. If women begin to function at a higher frequency, especially while pregnant, they can birth higher frequency children onto this planet. This massive shift can begin by simply changing our diets.

All the professionals mentioned thus far have created excellent plans to help restore the system through a healthy diet. Though slightly different in which foods they included, all their programs are similar. First you must eliminate the toxins in your body through a healthy diet and replenish the system with the right supplements and nutrition. I have personally completed Dr. Junger's Clean Program countless times and cannot begin to explain how it increased my health, wellbeing, and the shape of my body. The program is twenty-one days of clean eating through shakes and supplements with one healthy meal midday. The program helps people become clear on their toxic triggers and allows individuals to remove and rotate foods when they are done. By reintroducing foods slowly after a diet-cleanse, it is easy to identify what the body reacts to. I found it simpler to make these changes through a program; however, this can be done on your own. When I began to eat clean and take the right nutritional supplements, my skin became clear, my mind fog lifted, my energy increased, and I felt happy. Once you commit to wellbeing there is no going back to the way it was before.

Note to the reader: It is especially powerful to detox and replenish the body in order to prepare for conception and keep your family healthy. You should not do a deep intentional detox within six weeks of getting pregnant or a heavy metal detox within three months of getting pregnant to avoid affecting the baby. Optimally create a detox plan and healthy eating lifestyle six months to a year before conception. When you are pregnant please consult your doctor on how to maintain your clean lifestyle while still receiving the amount of nutrients needed to sustain your growing fetus. Children in your family should also eat clean, but refer to your pediatrician before providing any supplements. This applies to pregnancy also.

LET'S CLEAN UP YOUR DIET—HERE IS A PLAN

Dairy: Get off it and stop dairy foods. Dairy bogs down the liver, prevents toxins from leaving your body, and can create a heightened allergic state in your body. If you really need it and want an alternative, switch to goat cheese or yogurt.

Grains and High Glycemic Foods: Eat a low glycemic diet to stabilize your hormone levels. High glycemic foods cause an increase in inflammatory chemicals, stress, fluid retention, headaches, and insomnia. Stop all products containing gluten (wheat, barley, or rye) and refined carbohydrates (cookies, chips, and crackers). Grains are a modern-day discovery, and our systems are not adapted to process them. If you choose to include grains, go for healthy alternatives such as brown rice, buckwheat, millet, and quinoa.

Beans, lentils, legumes: Limit to one cup per day as they are difficult for most people to digest. Soak them before you cook them.

Sugar: Eliminate. No soft drinks and no artificial sweeteners. Studies show that mice that were addicted to cocaine and then offered sugar as an alternative will choose the sugar one hundred percent of the time!

Caffeine: If you can, get off it; if not, limit it.

Canola Oil: Damaging to the immune system, feeds the bad pathogens in your body, and eats away at the linings of your body.

Corn and Soy: Eliminate corn and soy products because they tend to be allergens, and because they are genetically modified, the altered DNA feeds the bad bacteria in the gut leading to chronic illness. If you find this difficult, try eliminating them for a couple of weeks and reintroducing to see what effect they have on your energy level.

WHAT YOU WANT TO EAT

Fats and Protein: Make sure to eat good fats: Omega-3 rich foods (such as wild caught salmon), avocados, nuts (No peanuts because of allergies.), and coconut oil. Avoid vegetable oils. Nuts and seeds are a good source of healthy fats and proteins (Try soaking them for easier digestion.).

Vegetables and Fruits: We co-evolved with plants, not with animals. Eat nutrient-dense, organic, and chemical-free fruits and vegetables. Include a lot of kale, collards, and mustard greens. It is ideal to have your diet be sixty to seventy percent fruits and vegetables. Villoldo explained, "A plant-based diet (nutrient-dense, calorie-poor) will switch on more than five hundred genes that create health and switch off more than two hundred genes that create cancers."

Meat: Eat sparingly and only free-range or grass-fed.

Fish: Eat small, wild caught Fish. Watch out for mercury toxicity.

Eggs: Great for you, if you are not allergic. Look for organic, free-range, pasture-raised eggs because they are higher in Omega-3 and vitamins A and E. Eggs are a great source of protein, and they don't affect cholesterol.

OPTIONAL SUPPLEMENTS

We take herbs or supplements to maintain the same frequency of the plant so that your health won't fall below that. The herbs have a specific vibration, and when you take them daily over a long period of time, your health can stay at the same base vibration of the plant. If you take ginseng daily for the rest of your life, you will maintain that level of vitality in your body because the supplement carries a specific quality and a high amount of energy. I personally think that everyone should take a multivitamin daily, but everyone needs to feel what their body needs beyond that. This book provides a lot of information, and the last thing I want you to feel is that you aren't doing enough or start to overcompensate; pick the things that work for you. Most importantly, pick the herbs or supplements that work for you, and if you need help doing this visit a naturopath, herbalist, or Chinese medicine doctor for advice.

The following is a list of supplements taken from Dr. Christian Northrup's Master Program and Albert Villoldo's One Spirit Medicine. I included an explanation of a handful of different supplements so that you understand what they do and why people may choose them. You have to decide what is right for you and can go to each of their individual programs for more guidance on dosing and maintenance. There is also a significant number of herbs that benefit health, which is too much for the breadth of this book. I encourage you to find the supplements or herbs that energetically feel right for your body. It is not about quantity but quality. A high-quality vitamin and mineral should be taken daily, especially if you are not eating enough fruits and vegetables.

Vitamin A: Helps to regulate excessive estrogen levels.

Vitamin B12: Essential for liver detoxification and for protecting DNA. Most of us are B12 deficient. Be sure to take sublingual methylcobalamin, an enhanced form of B12 that dissolves quickly under the tongue.

Vitamin C: Essential for detoxification processes.

Vitamin D3: Can prevent or reduce depression, dementia, diabetes, and autoimmune disorders.

Folic Acid: Protects the baby's neural tube development. Dosing is dependent on preexisting conditions, and you may need to speak to your doctor to ensure you are getting enough. 400 mcg daily is the average daily dose.

Iodine: A trace element that improves cognition, metabolism, protects the thyroid, and balances hormones. It is necessary for optimal health of the breasts, ovaries, and uterus.

S-acetyl glutathione: The first truly bioavailable form of the free-radical scavenger glutathione.

DHA and EPA: Omega-3 fatty acids important for brain health and preventing Alzheimer's. Take this in plant-based form.

Curcumin: The active ingredient in the spice turmeric activates the genes that turn on powerful antioxidants in the brain.

Trans-resveratrol: Triggers production of the brain's antioxidants and down-regulates genes that activate apoptosis, programmed cell death.

Pterostilbene: Found in blueberries and grapes. Works with trans-resveratrol to prevent cancer and other diseases.

Probiotic: Creates healthy flora in the gut and facilitates digestion.

Alpha-lipoic acid: Helps eliminate toxins and heavy metals in brain tissue.

Magnesium Citrate: Helps with your bowel movement and to eliminate waste, as well as relax your muscles.

Note to the Reader: The above supplements were chosen because they power up the brain. Anthony William, author of Medical Medium, introduced readers across the world to a list of foods and supplements that can help heal specifically heavy metal toxicity, viral illness, thyroid imbalances, and many other diseases. His recommendations are incredibly valuable but too detailed for the breadth of this book. Please refer to his resource for more information. He has helped many women with fertility and pregnancy. Also refer to the next section of this book for supplements that should be taken during pregnancy. This information is not to replace advice from your licensed medical practitioner.

4. OVERCOMING FOOD ADDICTIONS AND DISORDERS

"In order to change we must be sick and tired of being sick and tired."

–UNKNOWN

I personally struggled with an eating disorder for many years. It started when I was around the age of sixteen while living in a dysfunctional family situation. I used binging on foods and purging to maintain a sense of internal control over my chaotic environment. At my worst, I was doing this several times daily in my teenage years. In between these episodes, I hardly allowed myself to eat a single item with any nutritional value. The disorder left me emotionally and physically exhausted. I was depleted, swollen from fluid imbalance, desperate, and unhappy. Carbohydrates, sugars, and an inner need for peace were all triggers. Once I had a bite, the guilt was too heavy, so I just kept going and would often consume much more than the normal person could. I would then take relief in the bathroom and leave with bloodshot eyes and deep shame.

Many women share this story, and it took me long time to heal, as it does for everyone. There is hardly a single woman I know who does not look at their body and want to change something about it. We live in a society where it is accepted to think we are not enough, and lack of self-love is rampant. The best way to weaken the strongest group of people on the planet is to make them hate themselves through propaganda and massive advertisements from the time that they can understand English. The thought form that we are not good enough has been programmed into our subconscious from the time we are in the womb onward. Our mothers, commercials, books, and mass media all portray an image that distorts our view of reality of what we should look like. This is an even greater concern for upcoming generations as a result of social media platforms and the high use of technology. I personally had to peel away a lot of levels and go deep into my subconscious to conquer the beast within. The Western approach of cognitive therapy and an antidepressant didn't work for me. It was my deep dive into Spirit and Kundalini Yoga and Meditation that finally stopped the cycle and completely healed this disorder. The experience left me with a healthier approach to food, more balance, and a deep understanding of how hard it is to change our habits.

A teacher once said that ninety percent of women have eating disorders. I doubt that this statistic can be scientifically proven, but I personally agree. As a culture, women especially have an unhealthy relationship with food. We either consume too much or too little, and our identity to our weight and shape tends to be negative. Abraham Maslow made it clear that any individual who thinks he or she is hungry may be craving comfort, dependence, or vitamins. Food is interlocked with emotions, and eating healthy can create internal homeostasis. Until there is an emotional balance with food and a healthy connection, it will be very difficult for a person to move up the hierarchy of needs because issues won't be satisfied, and there will always be an emotional or physical craving of some sort. Many people are unaware of their issues with food or cover it up through a controlled and limited diet. Even if we heal our obsession with food, we often transfer our neurotic and habitual patterns to some new area of our lives. I do not want you to limit your consumption of food because of fear. I just want you to slowly peel back your layers so that you can shine your light.

There is a lot of shame around weight and staying healthy, and we often put a heavy burden on ourselves by trying to give up everything we love all at once. When we go all in, many of us fail, which fills us with more guilt, shame, and insecurity. These are the emotions we are trying to rise above in the first place. The goal is not to feel pain and suffering every second. We are aiming to rise above our bad habits and addictions through a balanced approach to all parts of life. As a culture, we must heal our issues surrounding food and body image so that we don't pass these problems on to our children during pregnancy. Most importantly, women must heal so that they can feel comfortable eating a healthy diet and manage the changes their body goes through with joy.

There are some clear signs that you may be addicted to certain foods including an unhealthy attachment, binge eating, or hiding your eating habits. Liana Werner-Gray, author of the *Earth Diet: Your Complete Guide to Living Using Earth's Natural Ingredients*, made herself sick from her addiction to junk foods. Her habit included starving herself for days and then overindulging on unhealthy foods for long periods of time, which would make her crash. She did this for five years until she wound up in the hospital. You can learn from people's personal stories so that you don't have to wait to get sick to make a change in your lifestyle.

To switch her life around, she committed to living off only foods from the earth for a year, and this radically changed her life and thousands of others. Rather than believing she was on a diet, she began to think of her changes as a lifestyle upgrade that increased her vibrational frequency, health, and happiness. It also reconnected her back to Spirit and the Earth, and she went directly to the land for her food. Her approach managed to get her out of her vicious eating cycle because she was committed to her health, but she still ate foods that she loved. Werner-Grey focused on alternating foods with healthier choices. She still ate chocolate, but she created her own healthy recipes with nutrient-dense replacements, such as creating chocolate balls primarily from nuts and cocoa nibs. This is something you to could adapt. Perhaps you like gummy bears; try buying them corn syrup free instead! Every little choice matters.

When you begin this process, choose one thing that you can eliminate. Pick your biggest obstacle and replace that one first. For example, if you love pizza, replace it with a gluten-free and organic pizza. One upgrade can lead to another. We want to give your body what it craves because you all have innate wisdom to know what is best for yourself. However, it is important that the body begins to crave healthier earth-based food choices. When you begin to choose better food replacements, your taste buds will change over time. Eventually, the junk food you once loved will not resonate with you because your cells will be different, and you will no longer crave the lower vibrational foods.

EXERCISE:

Use the following tools to help you overcome addictions: Visualize your dream body. It can be light, free, incredibly joyful, agile, flexible, healthy, or fun. Hold the vision as much as possible during the day, and consistently repeat self-affirming and positive words to yourself. Do it while walking, exercising, and cooking. This creates new neural pathways in your brain. Positive visualizations and personal mantras increase our self-worth and are proven ways to live a life without limits and full of health. Another way to begin to gain self-love and acceptance is staring at your body naked in the mirror for eleven minutes a day and praising yourself. Commit to do this for forty days and see the changes you will make!

MEDITATION FOR HEALING ADDICTIONS AS TAUGHT BY YOGI BHAJAN

Yogi Bhajan said that the medical effects and benefit of this meditation will not be fully understood for five hundred years. Imbalance is a modern epidemic, and this meditation helps to activate the brain areas to heal addictions that were thought to be unbreakable.

Posture: Sit in an Easy Pose with legs crossed and straight spine.

Mudra: Make fists of both hands and extend the thumbs straight. Place the thumbs on the temples and find the niche where the thumbs just fit.

Meditation: Lock the back molars together and keep the lips closed. Keeping the teeth pressed together throughout, alternately squeeze the molars tightly and then release the pressure. A muscle will move in rhythm under the thumbs. Feel it massage the thumbs and apply a firm pressure with the hands.

Eyes: Should remain closed and focused at the spot between the eyebrows. Silently vibrate Sa-Ta-Na-Ma at the brow with each squeeze of the molars. Complete for five to seven minutes.

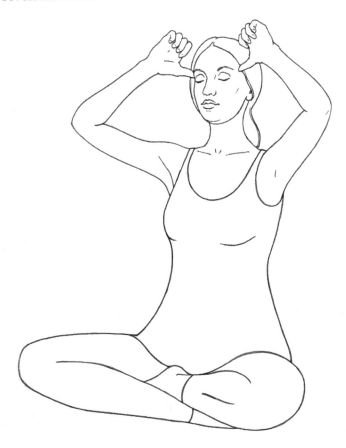

5. TAKE TIME OUT FOR
YOUR FOOD

"We have to bring children into a new relationship to food that connects them to culture and agriculture."

−ALICE WATERS

When you begin to change your diet to be more plant-based form, you will ultimately connect to the subtle energies of the earth and eating will become a more spiritual experience. To have a deeper connection to your food, always consider how you are feeling when you are eating, which will help you to see if you are working from your limbic system or your neocortex. If you are frantic or stressed, you are probably shoving carbs into your mouth and reacting from your limbic system. When your children are screaming, it is easy to hand them the fastest thing you can find to calm them down, which will most likely be processed foods to satiate their limbic brains. However, I encourage you to slow down and even prepare your meals ahead of time if necessary so that you have healthy options on hand. When you begin to pay attention to your emotions, you will have a better understanding of what you are eating and why. There are certain behaviors surrounding food that will help your family to have a better experience and a deeper to connection to what goes into your bodies.

The first step to connecting to the spiritual and emotional aspect of food is to eat it slowly. When you are eating, begin to pause to taste the subtle qualities of your food and feel the texture. This is what life is all about—the slow flow. Eating should not involve the conversations going on around you during every meal—nor should it be done while standing up, which is the typical mom stance. If you are eating fast, you are likely emotionally upset or in your head thinking too much. Children don't respond to what we say; they respond to how we act, and our behavior around cooking and eating can change the way they approach this vital aspect of life. We must teach them healthy behaviors surrounding food.

Chewing is an important action, and when done properly has a vast amount of health benefits for our bodies. It is interesting that we never grew up learning how to properly chew our food down to almost a liquid form for best digestion. Teaching children how to chew should be a course in itself. This is because chewing your food completely allows your energy to go elsewhere in your body and not solely to digestion. Another important behavior is to admire the colors on your plate to see if they are vibrant, beautiful, and varied. This is because the colors equate to energy, and our aim here is to make your body a stronger energetic system.

The preparation of your food can be a meditative art form, and altering the way you approach cooking can be fun. Use the ingredients, method, and visual presentation to create deep soul fulfillment and increase your life-force. What you eat can uplift you or decrease your energy, and it is time to commit to changing behaviors now so that the next generation can benefit from your willingness to heal yourself and your family through food. Even the act of cooking can be made into the most meditative of practices. The movements of your hands, your breath, and the placement of your instruments all becomes a small dance of creating internal balance through higher vibratory food and actions. Enriching your food with blessing is an uplifting way to live in line with Spirit as it allows you to connect. Children love these small acts of thankfulness. When you resonate with grace and joy, they will follow suite.

Another behavior to consider surrounding food is whether you eat together as a family or spread out around the house. We have forgotten the art of gathering around an actual table rather than a television. When you eat as a family, make sure the time at the table is like a holy temple of joy and laughter. Invite your neighbors over to enjoy your space and the food you have created to bless the group. Serving others in such a simple way can create more happiness in your life and is a great example for your children. One of the greatest acts of rebellion is just being nice to other people. Day-to-day gestures of kindness and giving are what will keep you moving forward on the path to brighter light.

EXERCISE:

When you start to change your diet, reflect on the following questions in a diary: How are you feeling when you choose your food? When you hold the food or beverage and look at it before eating or drinking, does it energetically match the frequency that you are trying to create? Does it taste sweet or sour, and how will that affect your demeanor? Is it dense or soft? Do you tend to eat heavier foods, such as burgers or fries when your mind is full of negative thoughts? When you are feeling your best, what are you eating? Is it light, vibrant, fragrant, and full of life?

6. CHANGE YOUR SLEEPING PATTERN FOR HIGHER WELLBEING

"The morning breeze has secrets to tell you, do not go back to sleep, do not go back to sleep, do not go back to sleep."

–RUMI

Sleep is a physiological need and required within the hierarchy for wellbeing. I am going to approach this basic need in a way that you may have never heard of before and explain how you can alter your sleep in a specific manner, or wake in the early mornings to meditate, in order to reach higher peaks of consciousness. Sleep is more than just a time of rest and change in brain wave functions as scientists have led us to believe. It is a time when humanity can connect to a higher source and many other dimensions of possibility other than this physical plane we call Earth. When you go to sleep, you are much more active than you are during the daytime because you are connecting to your God spark, but you just don't remember. In *Seth Speaks: The Eternal Validity of the Soul*, Jane Roberts explained that while sleeping you can travel out of your body and come into communication with other parts of your identity and with many other realities in the Universe. Sleep is a time when you are learning, studying, and playing on a Spiritual level. Though it seems that you are unconscious, this is far from the case. There are many reasons why our waking and sleeping hours are so disconnected and we cannot remember what happens at night. One of the main problems is the belief that we need long blocks of time sleeping, rather than shorter periods.

Sleeping in two shorter increments seems very natural to me as it allows for more short bursts of energy throughout the day and offers the opportunity to remember what happened during our dreamtime. Roberts explained that men in Paleolithic times always slept in short bursts because of hunting and daylight. The human adaptation of dividing time in two long blocks of sleeping and waking consciousness is an ingrained societal pattern that may have occurred historically when individuals moved into dwellings over time. Years ago, if someone told me to sleep less than eight hours, I would have called them nuts, as you may be doing now to me. As a mother, or soon-to-be mother, you may feel that this is a ridiculous idea and that sleep is the most precious time of the day. Stick with me on this theory though; let's see how we can help you to create a sleep time patterning that connects you deeper to yourself in order to become a more creative and focused parent. This theory, just like cleansing your body of toxins, should not be done while pregnant or breastfeeding because during this time you need to rest for longer periods.

According to Roberts, to recuperate, regenerate, and connect to ourselves deeper, we must reduce our sleep to around a five-hour block with a nap later if needed. Too much sleep, such as ten hours at a time, causes the body to become sluggish. Just as having light snacks throughout the day rather than three heavy meals can make you feel lighter and more in touch, reducing our sleep into two smaller blocks over twenty-four hours will positively affect our body, mind, and spirit. More frequent and briefer periods of sleep will cause you to have higher peaks of conscious focus and increased physical and psychic ability. Sleeping eight to ten hours straight creates a great division in yourself, because your spirit is literally disconnected from the body for too long of a period. It is instead ideal to sleep in five-hour blocks of time, and if you require more sleep, you could take a long nap up to two hours. Other people may benefit from a four-hour block of sleep followed by two naps.

You may be thinking how is this possible if I hold a job with normal working hours or I have children? I recommend that you sleep between four to six hours at night and take a nap or rest when you get home from work after you eat. When you wake early in the morning, you will find that these hours are full of great creativity and an opportunity to complete tasks that you normally wouldn't have time for during the day, such as meditating. I once held the belief system that I absolutely required eight hours of sleep straight and was always the first to go home at night. Over time, as I questioned my beliefs, I found that if I reduced my amount of sleep and woke in the early morning hours to meditate or write, I functioned at a much higher level the rest of the day. Sometimes I needed a short nap later, but overall, I still felt better. Rising in the early hours before sunrise after around six hours of sleep helps me to maintain an incredibly high vibration full of enthusiasm that everyone around me can feel too. Some days I do need eight straight hours of sleep, and I always trust my body.

If you feel that you absolutely always need eight to nine hours of sleep, that is fine; the most important concept that you need to take from this section is the importance of setting a time of day to meditate and be with yourself before conception, during pregnancy, and into motherhood. This is one of the most important points in the entire book, and if you commit to it, this time will change your life and your children's lives. The early morning provides the best opportunity to meditate because of the way the sun hits the earth, and it also sets the day in motion to feel more joy. When I switched to sleeping in these blocks of time, I saw a significant increase in my ability to function, creative capabilities, and focus. In the morning hours, I meditate and I write because this period of time is bursting with energy for me, and I often accomplish more before nine AM than the average person accomplishes by six PM.

This change was not immediate, and it took me up to a year to really be able to alter this habit that is so ingrained in our society. It started when I was introduced to the concept and lifestyle of Kundalini Yoga and Meditation. Sadhana is a practice that many yogis across the world have been doing for thousands of years. Guru Singh wrote *21st Century Prophets The Sage Within* and described the science behind waking in the early mornings with the purpose of increasing your energy. He said, "There are two and a half hours before the rise of the sun, where the rays of arriving light are infrared. This is known to the Yogis and Masters as "amrit vela" the "ambrosial hours." This is a time when early light—it's an invisible light—carries vast quantities of information for nourishing life…These infrared rays are attuned to the longer "theta" waves of your dreamtime brain, which is the same state of the brain in deep meditation." The best activities to complete in the morning to create a higher frequency and more intuition are stretching, yoga poses, chanting mantras, silent meditations, deep breathing, or even just being grateful for the day to come.

As a mother, you can help to create a strong and safe foundation for your child, and ultimately create a thriving human being, through a daily meditation practice. Kundalini Yoga and Meditation, as taught by Yogi Bhajan, is the fastest growing yoga on the planet and also the fastest way to increase awareness. The meditations are generally active with movement and mantra, which makes them fun. Throughout this book, various Kundalini Meditations will be introduced that can be implemented into your daily practice. If you are new to meditation, it is better to meditate daily, even if it is short, compared to an occasional longer attempt. A daily practice of three to eleven minutes is a good place to start. With time you will find that you may want to increase your meditation period because of the pure joy and stability it brings.

The time upon waking is sacred because it sets the tone for the rest of your day. Waking in the morning to meditate sets the tone for a life of victory and trust in your own capabilities. If you can commit to waking up early every morning, you can accomplish anything; this I promise you. I started to get up early every morning when I was pregnant with my second child. At that point, I didn't know what I was doing or why, but I would compulsively rise to chant what is called the Long Ek Ong Kar in Kundalini Yoga. There are thousands of meditations to choose from, but this must have been what the baby wanted. I found out later that this is the best meditation to shift consciousness and bridge the gap between the mother and the child.

At first, naturally, it was hard to get up early and change my sleep cycle to be shorter at night. I could think of every excuse in the world at the time as to why it was a bad idea including the fact I was pregnant, tired, caring for a year-old child during the day, and still finishing my FNP degree. I started waking up to chant for thirty minutes, which turned into forty-five minutes, and eventually I meditated for up to two hours a morning. This may sound absolutely shocking to individuals who have never heard of such a thing, but what I know for sure is that spending time in the morning to meditate, even if it is just ten minutes, will significantly affect the amount that you accomplish during the day. If you cannot switch how many hours you sleep, the most important thing to do is get up in the morning and do something that makes you feel good so that you can carry that positive frequency into the rest of your day. You will become more effective, focused, and creative with your time.

Waking up in the morning to meditate is wonderful for mothers as it allows you time alone for self-love and grounding and demonstrates a commitment to increasing your happiness and connection to Spirit for the family. Now, I do not even have to set an alarm to wake up; my body naturally rises, and I am excited for this time. Shocking but true. The amount of time that I spend meditating in the morning often varies, and so do the meditations I complete, but I always do one meditation that is the same every day so that I can go deeply into it.

There are a variety of benefits to changing our sleep function including an upgrade in our physical, mental, creative, and psychic abilities. When our patterns of sleep are altered, we become less rigid and rigorous with our concept of time, which reduces our tendency to become neurotic over schedules. Life is a twenty-four hour clock. Do not limit yourself. When you experience this you can be free and gain your power back over the time space continuum. This will help you when you are awake at night with a newborn. Though this change is different from what doctors recommend, it will result in a greater understanding of the nature of the universe and of yourself. You will have more peak experiences throughout the day, times of insight, and a deeper connection to your world. Your concentration on tasks at work or at home will increase, your ability to make decisions will improve, and you will learn more efficiently. If you want to correctly interpret reality and have a bright, powerful, and uncluttered personality, you need to switch to shorter periods of rest rather than one long block of time sleeping or at least start a meditation practice.

EXERCISE:

Wake up just ten minutes earlier than normal to meditate, be grateful, breathe, or journal. Just start here and see where this takes you. Add more time as you begin to see a change in your demeanor and wellbeing. Use the meditations explained in this book as your starting point. Mindful breath is a simple but profound way to shift your perspective. Your mind follows your breath. The key to controlling your mind is controlling your breath.

BREATH EXERCISES YOU CAN BEGIN THE DAY WITH:

Sitali Pranayam: Curl the tongue into a "U" shape, inhale through the curled tongue, and exhale through the nose. Do this twenty-six times to reduce anger.

Long Deep Breathing: Using the full capacity of the lungs, inhale deeply and expand the abdomen, then the chest and the upper ribs, and clavicle. Exhale in reverse until the abdomen pulls in and up.

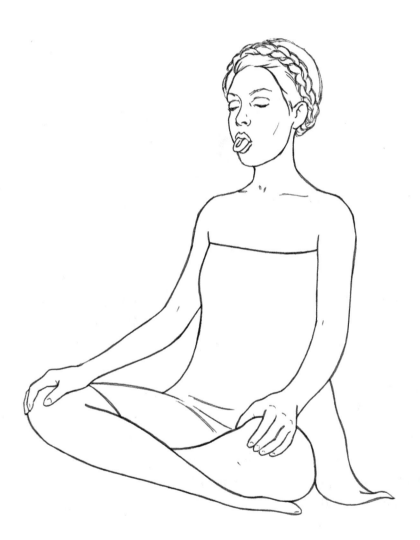

7. ENHANCING YOUR FERTILITY

"The jump is so frightening between where I am and where I want to be. Because of all I may become, I will close my eyes and leap.

—MARY ANNE RUDMACHER

Fertility is a delicate subject and like a flower needs to be discussed with care because when we want something so badly, and what we want does not come fast enough, there is an aching in our hearts that feels like we are being ripped open. When a woman is ready for a child, a gap grows in time and space, and the desire to hold the baby becomes the forefront of her thoughts. I have watched many friends battle with fertility issues and months pass with empty arms, more longing, less control, and a stronger desire for the outcome. I have also witnessed the unbearable loss of children in utero through my patients, which becomes a heavy burden of confusion after months of attempting to become pregnant. If you are trying to get pregnant and have become frustrated with the process, I don't have all the answers here, as fertility is one of the greatest mysteries of our time, but I have simple theories that may shed some light on the space you are feeling inside. I am going to provide you with ways to better connect to your womb through meditations and the energetics of food.

In ancient times, women's only focus as a young girl was bearing children, but in the modern day, we are blessed to spread our energy out in many directions.

Women now focus on going to school, working, traveling, or buying their own house and have entered this male-dominated world with vigor. Though reaching high levels of our masculine nature can be rewarding, it can also create a dichotomy in our fields that disconnects us from our wombs. Many women spend years focused on achieving their goals and energetically pushed the thought of bearing children out of their field, so when the time comes that they are ready to bear a child, their body, mind, and spirit have to align. Women often have to make up for lost time quickly if they choose to have a baby later in life. Females have to relate to time in completely different ways than males do when it comes to their physical body and having children.

Women who have tried to become pregnant for a significant amount of time, over one year, may be operating on a reproductive system that lacks energy. One of the main reasons for this could be a long period of time on birth control, which teaches the body to divert resources away from the reproductive system to energetically avoid conceiving. Birth control was an amazing and progressive finding in our society and women should absolutely under no circumstances have a baby until they are ready for the sake of the child and the mother. Yogi Bhajan said, "It is very essential for the woman to be very, very sensible because then only can she create in the child of tomorrow, the very manifestation to be a very sensible person." Birth control is important. Don't stop it until you are ready and willing to bring a child on to this planet. Just begin to connect to your womb and mentally, emotionally, and spiritually prepare yourself for the coming of your child long before you are ready to conceive. Your reproductive system is its own entity and has its own soul and life. Your womb requires conscious attention and nurturing to keep it connected to heaven.

The connection between birth control and a low battery reproductive system may not be the case for all women, but for some that have been on the pill or other forms of birth control for a significant amount of time, this may be the issue. Though drug companies and many doctors would disagree with this belief system, birth control teaches the body to withhold pregnancy for many years, creating an energetic pattern. When you are ready to get pregnant, you need to reconnect and charge the reproductive organs back up, a system that was probably not previously paid attention too. Women should always have the option of taking birth control but may need time to reconnect with this area of the body, that has been energetically drained, when they are ready to become pregnant.

Anthony William, author of *Medical Medium*, was provided the gift to speak with Spirit since childhood and has saved thousands of people's lives and improved their health through simple changes in their diet. He was the first person to discuss the need to energetically recharge the reproductive organs through meditation and food in a way that I and many other women could understand. In his book, *Life Changing Foods*, he discussed the four most detrimental environmental factors to our health and specific foods for increasing fertility. His plan is simple and easy to maintain, and I believe it is far ahead of its time in delivering the knowledge that women need in order to maintain their fertility in the coming years. Though the detrimental environmental factors, which William calls the unforgiving four, are not the focus of this section, they must be mentioned because they are significant to health and fertility. William said, "If you're looking to point fingers about how things got so bad in the world, here's where to look: radiation, toxic heavy metals, the viral explosion and DDT." These invisible intruders have wreaked havoc on our health for decades or longer and are passed down through family lines. Fruits and vegetables carry an energetic frequency that can help to heal these invaders in our system.

If you have been trying to conceive for quite some time and are unable to for no identifiable reason, there are some foods that you could try eliminating from your diet. William explained that it is important to avoid adrenalized foods from animals including chicken, turkey, lamb, and other types of meat, dairy, and fish. Adrenaline is an antifertility drug, and at the time of death, these animals are filled with it because of their fear response. Even trace amounts of animal products can have an energetic effect on your body. Stress should also be reduced as this emotion also affects the adrenals. When the body is putting a significant amount of energy into one area of your life, it cannot divert any energy to other places because the reserves are all taken up. Think about it this way: your body becomes incredibly tight and needs to relax. If you are suffering from adrenal fatigue, try eating small meals every one to two hours to prevent your adrenals from working overtime. If you are dealing with PCOS, endometriosis, PID, uterine fibroids, or cysts you want to avoid eating eggs, corn, wheat, canola oil, dairy, aspartame, MSG, and soy products. According to William, you also want to avoid phytotoxic hormone chemicals including pesticides, herbicides, and plastics as much as you can. Chlorine and fluoride should also be included in this list. Though there is a lot of things you should avoid to increase fertility, there is also a lot of things you can have that are very beneficial for your body that are listed below.

FERTILITY FOR WOMEN:

√ Fruit: William said, "Eat Fruit to Produce Fruit." This is very important. When you fill your body with high vibrational foods, the life-giving properties and energetics of the products become a part of you. The reproduction system runs on glucose, so rather than focus on a high-protein diet or a low-carb diet before pregnancy, focus on a natural glucose diet through organic fruit. Berries, especially wild blueberries, are excellent for balancing hormones. Other great fruits for fertility include: oranges, bananas, avocados, grapes, melons, mangoes cucumbers, limes, and cherries.

√ Foods that help bring change to the reproductive system (or if you have a history of PCOS, endometriosis, PID, uterine fibroids or cysts) include: artichokes, asparagus, spinach, kale, celery, butter leaf lettuce, garlic, potatoes, sprouts, coconut, microgreens, red clover, raspberry leaf, nettle leaf, and raw honey.

√   Celery Juice: Celery is a powerful anti-inflammatory because it starves the bad bacteria in your gut. Disease comes from an acidic body and green foods help to alkalize your system. Celery also helps to cleanse your body of toxic heavy metals. Drink sixteen ounces or more of fresh juice on an empty stomach upon rising daily.

√   Eggplant: According to Yogi Bhajan, eggplant is the best food a woman can eat for health and strength.

√   Vitamin E helps to boost fertility and is a natural antioxidant. Take up to 500 to 800 IU for a few months before conception as it helps the fertilized egg stay attached to the uterus.

√   Raspberry leaf tea: Drink this throughout the day. It helps to increase lactation turning on the system.

√   Eliminate chocolate of all kinds. It is caffeinated and full of toxic products. Don't eat this during pregnancy either.

√   Avoid all illegal drugs and alcohol.

FERTILITY FOR MEN:

√   Male Fertility: The same foods listed above will be very beneficial for men too. It is important that they reduce their toxic heavy metal loads too as mercury is one of the main causes of drops in fertility in males. The specific protocol for doing this is in Anthony William' books, and it includes incorporating Hawaiian Spirulina, frozen wild blueberries, cilantro, garlic, and barley grass juice into the diet. Other supplements that are helpful include: ashwagandha, zinc (for healthy sperm), red clover blossoms, and vitamin B12.

√   According to Yogi Bhajan, who was the master of Kundalini Yoga and Yogic Science, fresh figs with saffron milk promote vitality and prostate health for men. Soak one tablespoon saffron overnight in one-half cup milk (Any type of milk can be used.). In the morning, blend the milk and saffron until smooth. Wash ten to fifteen fresh figs. Draw milk and saffron into a clean syringe and inject the saffron "nectar" into the figs. Eat up to three per day and store the rest in the freezer.

√   Onions, ginger, and garlic are known as the trinity roots and are high potency foods for men. Yogi Bhajan taught that garlic increases semen in the body and provides higher sexual energy for the male.

√   Breakfast to overcome impotency: Yogi Bhajan taught that men should take milk, almonds, cardamom, and honey, and blend them together for breakfast and don't eat for four hours afterward.

√   If you can find it, banyan tree milk helps to regulate the semen and the testicles, creating high-potency sperm. Take six drops daily. Ghee, or unclarified butter, is also important to eat for sperm production according to Kundalini Yogic Science.

√   Men should not heavily drink or smoke marijuana (along with any other illegal drugs) especially while trying to conceive. If unable to stop, at least reduce the amount the week or two before ovulation.

MEDITATIONS AND ACTIONS TO BOOST FERTILITY

√   Walking Meditation: While walking, tell your womb that you are one hundred percent ready to conceive now and fully behind your decision. Honor your reproductive system not with demands but with respectful guidance. While walking, you can call upon the Angel of Fertility for additional support throughout your journey. Do this exercise daily to remain connected and give your system permission to become pregnant.

√ Breathing White Light: While lying on your back, take deep breathes into your abdomen, expanding up to your lungs. With each inhale, draw the white light into your womb. When you are doing this, you are taking the attention out of your head and directing the energy to another part of your body. Let your body know that it is now your sacred mission to become pregnant and you are fully ready to consciously bring a child into this world.

√ If you don't know what the reproductive system looks like, you might want to get a picture of it so that you can actually visualize how the egg and sperm come together during conception and feel this in your body.

√ Ovary massage: Helps to increase your vitality and connect to your reproductive organs. Do it in bed when you get up or with oil or in warm water for comfort. Find your pubic bone and then your hip bone and about equal distance in between you can locate your ovaries bilaterally. Do this for about five minutes, and you will really start to open up.

√ Parathyroid Massage: May help the thyroid to come into balance for your hormonal functioning. Open your eyes wide, grab the area under your chin, open your mouth, and say ahhh with a loud open mouth while gently shaking the area.

√ Make sure that you know when you are ovulating. You can buy simple home monitoring kits for this or use the temperature method. Do not let your male partner ejaculate a week before you make love, and his sperm will have a much higher ejaculation load. Over-ejaculation causes depletion of the vitality of the sperm and can deplete the man's energy. Male sperm should be the consistency of yogurt; if it is less than this, his energy is low according to Yogi Bhajan.

√ Make sure both you and your partner go to a health practitioner for a full checkup before you conceive.

√ Acupuncture combined with herbal medicine will benefit your whole system.

√ When there is tension around the reproductive organs, energy can't flow as well. When you are trying to get pregnant, do not wear tight underwear or pants. Massage the lymph around your pelvis and lower legs. Keep the circulation flowing to this area through mental and physical acts.

√ If you often get urinary tract infections after sex, try using coconut oil as a lubricant before sex.

√ In order to maintain a balanced pH in the vaginal canal, you can douche with organic yogurt mixed with a couple drops of tea tree oil three days before and three days after your period. Use ten parts water and one part yogurt mixed together. When you are menstruating, don't put pressure in the pelvic area or lift anything heavy. Reduce your exertion to maintain high energy levels.

√ You may need to adjust your weight before pregnancy for fertility. Some people may need to lose weight, and others may need to gain weight. Eating fruit and vegetables with proper exercise can help you do this or completing what Yogi Bhajan called the "Green Diet" will also balance your weight out. This diet consists of eating only green healthy items for forty days.

√   Maya abdominal massage, or deep tissue massage, treats infertility as well as other reproductive and pelvic disorders. It is a technique from Central America.

ANDAJ KRIYA AS TAUGHT BY YOGI BHAJAN

This meditation helps to adjust the ovaries in women, which will assist with conception. Yogi Bhajan said, "You want your kidneys and ovaries to become balanced? Just balance your hands straight before you. Don't do anything else. Am I asking you to meditate or do anything? No. Just don't be irritated. That's all I'm saying. Don't react. You will react. Yes, yes. The ovaries are getting adjusted. And if the egg has been released by the wrong ovary, you will find a surprise in your body. You have to adjust your ovaries every month, and there's no other way other than the Andaj kriya. There's no other kriya which can do it. This is the elbow and this is ninety degrees, absolutely parallel. It automatically stretches the body and the entire area and the action and reaction will balance. Remember when you had an ovarian cyst, and what it cost with all the insurance?"

Posture: Sit with a straight spine. Stretch the arms out in front of you. Before each Kundalini mediation you can tune in by chanting "Ong Namo Guru Dev Namo" three times in order to connect to yourself and to all the Masters that came before you. Bend the elbows so the forearms are ninety degrees straight up, the upper arms parallel to the floor. Palms are flat and face one another, held at the level of the top of the head. The fingers point up. Lift the diaphragm. Note: The elbow to fingers should be straight up at a ninety-degree angle. Not right, not left. Straight up. "Two ninety-degree angles."

Mantra: Sing along with a tape such as "I am bountiful." (This can be found on YouTube.). You can sing: I Am Bountiful, Blissful, and Beautiful. Bountiful, Blissful, and Beautiful I am, or Bountiful am I, Blissful am I, Beautiful am I.

Time: Practice up to 31 minutes. Start with 3 to 11 minutes and work your way up.

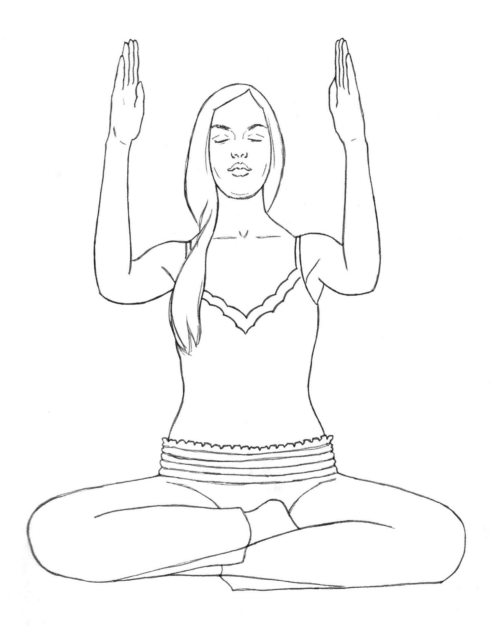

8. PREPARATION FOR CONSCIOUS CONCEPTION

"The coming children in 90 years from today will have a brain with a special development around the point of the pineal gland. They will have small cells which shall be known by the knowledgeable people as vibratory centers through which ordinary men shall communicate at long distance at the same time without physical, with their psyches and shall have effect and the reverse effect of all the knowledge of the mental process at different frequencies to relate to that great human vibratory level on which the future consciousness man shall talk and communicate. I am making a statement. You can mark it down."

–YOGI BHAJAN 1972

The most important concepts you must understand regarding conscious conception is that it takes a significant amount of mental, emotional, and spiritual preparation and that pregnancy is something you should absolutely not take on if you are not fully ready. People all over the world are procreating, but as we can see, not much has improved. This is why conscious conception is so important, and if you are reading this and prepared to do the work, you could change the planet. Throughout this book, I will refer to the male and female "partnership" when it comes to creating and raising a child because essentially that's the base equation needed to produce, but I understand that families are made up of all sorts of equations. I am speaking to the single moms, split families, grandmothers, aunts, and fathers at different points throughout the text too as there are many ways to raise a child, and everyone needs to be on board. Conception requires just an ovum and a sperm, but if you want to do it consciously, and you are ready to bring a high vibrational Being on to this planet, I am here to discuss some things that should have been put into mass consumption years ago.

As a conscious and prepared woman, you need to be ready and not take the responsibility or bringing a life into this world lightly. Yogi Bhajan said,

> *"It is absolutely wrong to be pregnant when you are spiritually, mentally, emotionally, or physically unprepared. It has been estimated that in a very fast society, eighty percent of all conceptions happen by chance... It is a very sad situation. To be very frank and honest, it will ruin the IQ of the child up to thirty-three percent. One-third of the possible IQ of the child, his potential health, his faculty of creativity, and his intelligence to deal with his personal security will be ruined if the mother was physically, mentally, and spiritually unprepared to conceive the child, and it will be a loss of another twenty percent if the father is similarly unprepared. Before it happens, the pregnancy should be totally, emotionally, characteristically, analytically, materially, physically, mentally, and spiritually discussed, planned, and noted down."*

If we want smart, creative, and resourceful leaders on earth, we need to prepare ourselves to produce and raise them properly without intruding on their own individuality. If you are ready to consciously conceive, you cannot begin to plan the pregnancy or call in the soul too early. Use your intention and prayer to plan your pregnancy for a very long time before you create the child in your womb. The planning and focused intention begins the moment you get the feeling you are ready or even in your teens if you know in the distant future you want children. Ancient Yogis would prepare for years and even lifetimes to bring an advanced soul into this world. It is best if you can prepare anywhere from three months to three years before conception, but if you don't have this amount of time, start right now. During this period, you will begin to create a relationship with the type of soul you want to bring down and intimately communicate with the Being by getting to know one another.

Just like you would pray to Spirit or God, you begin to connect with your baby long before you meet through open conversation and asking for the type of individual you would like to create. According to Gurujas, teacher at RAMA Institute and a world-renowned meditation teacher and music artist, the more that you meditate and pray on that specific soul, the higher caliber of soul you are going to bring down. Be specific and ask for the type of individual you want to conceive, and include your partner in this process if he is willing. Speak to the Universe with the intention of bringing in a sacred child and committing to your part of the process. Conscious conception also requires a daily practice of meditation and prayer. Kundalini Yoga Kriyas, which are yogic posture sets, can also help to get your glandular system running correctly. Many of the meditations in this book would be an excellent way to begin creating your daily meditation practice. I recommend starting with the Kirtan Kriya explained further in the book because of the great amount of benefit this meditation holds and the fact that it helps to regulate the menstrual cycle. Before conception, you also want to begin to speak with your partner about all the practicalities of raising a child before he or she actually arrives.

While it is important to spiritually and mentally prepare before you conceive a child, it is also vital to practically prepare with earthly concerns. Before you become pregnant, it is optimal to discuss the basic physiological, safety, and love needs that the child will require to grow consciously. It is a good idea to sit down with your partner and discuss all the details over a long period of time.

√   You need to fully understand what types of roles you and other family members will play. Will family members take care of your children?

√   Who will work and how many hours a week?

√   Which partner's career leads when it comes to taking care of children?

√   Do you agree on diet or even vaccinations?

√   What are your monetary fears and how will you feed and shelter the child?

√   What type of school do you hope the child will attend?

√   How do you plan to discipline?

√   Where will the child sleep?

√   Where do you ultimately want to live?

Personally, I never did any of this planning, and I wish from the bottom of my heart that I would have known better. That is why I am so dedicated to getting this material to you so that you can save yourself and your children simple worries that could be easily avoided. I can tell you from experience that you and your partner will not agree on everything after the child is born, and it can be a very stressful time. Hormones become imbalanced and emotions run deep when a baby arrives, and in the first years of child raising, it would be ideal for families to have a set of values to fall back on. When our first daughter arrived, I assumed that family members would step in and help us care for her, at least part of the time, which would have given me more freedom. This never happened, and it was heartbreaking, but it should have been something I discussed with them beforehand so that I did not set my expectations too high. My partner and I also did not set any clear expectations on what roles we would play when our babies were born or how long he would take leave from work. When he had to return to his company and long work hours, I was not prepared for his absence, and it shocked me, which only created blame and unnecessary guilt for him. If you are reading this and have not had your baby yet, much of your preparation can be done from the material supplied further in this book.

Beyond discussing the basic needs a family requires, you also need to get to know yourself deeply before having a baby, and even more importantly, you need to like yourself. If you want to conceive and birth a compassionate and loving child, you must love yourself first. If your self-esteem is low and you have not dealt with your personal insecurities or relationship issues, you will undoubtedly attract and create a child with a similar frequency and similar problems. Women have to go inside and discover all of the places that they are uncomfortable with and deal with the unresolved issues before they become pregnant so that these do not arise during motherhood, because I can promise you that they will. The meditations in this book are a great way to build the courage to have a child and will provide you a way to work through emotions. When you begin to connect to yourself, you will also begin to ultimately connect to the Infinite because you will realize that there is no difference. With your prayers come the answers; listen and you shall receive what you want in perfect timing. Let Mother Nature bring you what you want. Always know that everything happens just the way it is supposed to happen and in perfect timing. Learn to receive the great abundance.

EXERCISE:

According to Tej Khalsa, world-renowned yoga teacher and main author of the *Creating the Aquarian Child Manual*, before you have a baby, you need to take a personality inventory. This means that you must go through your personality and everything that happened to you up until now that brought you to where you are. Identify who you are as a mother, as a child, as a woman, and the impressions that other people put into you. Understand what you think a parent is and how you would act as one. Go through your memory bank and history—write it down and journal out your life. Consciously replace old memories with new ones. When you play old negative scenes, begin to create new memories over them by creating new mental projections that are more positive. Understanding your personality and history will help you to understand yourself.

GURPRASAAD MEDITATION AS TAUGHT BY
YOGI BHAJAN

"Just let it happen—health, wealth, happiness, your caliber, capacity. Fill your heart, fill your soul with whatever comes from the nature. This meditation is very restful. The pressure on the meridian points on the ribcage gives immediate relaxation."

–YOGI BHAJAN

Gurprasaad is a meditation for prayer, prosperity, and receiving.

Mudra: Sitting in Easy Pose with legs crossed, cup the hands in front of the heart center, palms side by side, face up, as if asking for a blessing.

Arms: Bring the arms into the chest so they rest on the rib cage. Begin with the eyes ninety percent closed, and allow them to close completely.

Mantra: None specified. Mentally recite any mantra you choose. Meditate on a specific intention and feel a deep inflow. A mantra is listed below or you could recite "I am Woman."

Time: This meditation can be practiced for any length of time. Start with eleven minutes and work up to thirty-one over time.

Note: You can play the following mantra, to add power to your prayer. Ardaas Bhaee can be found on YouTube. Any mantra that you like would work though.

"Ardaas Bhaee, Amar Daas Guroo, Amar Daas Guroo, Ardaas Bhaee. Raam Daas Guroo, Raam Daas Guroo, Raam Daas Guroo Sachee Sahee."

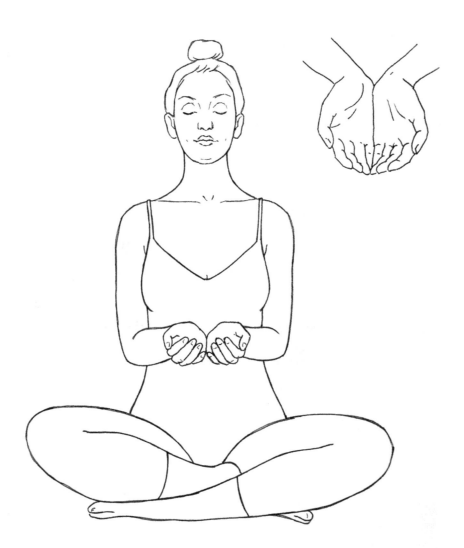

9. THE ART OF CONSCIOUS CONCEPTION THROUGH SEX OR FERTILITY TREATMENTS

"That is why, if the house is spiritual, then man enters a temple and then is a relationship of a devotee and a priestess. If you can create those hypnoses in the house, your man will never look out of the window, doesn't matter what. All men want a priestess, fairies and Goddesses but they will never ever admit it."

–YOGI BHAJAN

Conscious conception involves preparing your body for intercourse and generating a great amount of internal energy for expansion of the auric field. Today when couples have sex, it is typically unplanned and followed by a heavy dinner and drinks, which is the exact opposite of how things should occur if you are intending to do this mindfully. For most couples, intercourse is usually short and does not lead up to the degree of pleasure that should be happening between two people. For the sake of ease, I will be discussing sex between a man and a woman here, but please have full understanding that this connection can happen between same sex couples too. Guru Jagat, teacher in the *Creating the Aquarian Child Course* and author of *Invincible Living*, explained that intercourse, when completed the yogic way, is an act of self-worship where two bodies become one temple. If you are interested in conscious conception, I am going to provide a few simple steps that you can take before the time of ovulation to optimize the event in the hopes of conceiving. When you amplify your auric field and create a higher frequency, you have a better possibility of conceiving a child who can match that frequency or increase it.

Infertility over the next half a decade is estimated to rise significantly, and there will be an increase in the use of technology to conceive children. Though prediction rates are hard to prove until they occur, some sources claim that within forty years infertility will rise to an estimated fifty percent. This is why keeping connected to your womb, avoiding toxins, eating healthy foods, and aligning to Spirit and your baby long before you have a child is important. The subject is not being discussed enough, which is why this text is so significant. By preparing our bodies physically, emotionally, and spiritually, we will be more likely to bring life onto the planet in a conscious manner. The technology that is available to help couples that cannot conceive is a beautiful thing. These individuals can prepare for the event in a similar manner described in this section by creating a deep connection together and within. No matter how you conceive, by planning before the event, you can help to activate the process through your intent.

THE SEVENTY-TWO-HOUR WINDOW

Before conception, you must build a significant amount of energy and self-love. Conscious sexual encounters take more planning than the type of sexual experiences that we are typically used to in the western world. To begin, you must know when you are ovulating and create a seventy-two-hour window to amplify yourself before the actual event. In the case of receiving IVF, don't hesitate to increase your body energy in a similar manner three days before. If you are really interested in bringing down a powerful soul, and you have the patience and the time to wait for the right date, you could visit an advanced astrologer to specify the best times to conceive. It is best if both the female and the male increase their energy, but if your partner is not interested in conscious conception, that is fine. Focus on increasing your auric field, also known as the energetic body, through long deep breathing, breath of fire, chanting, meditation, long walks, or baths. When you are trying to conceive, both you and your partner should avoid alcohol and any other drugs. Your partner should also avoid ejaculating up to a week before you are ovulating to increase the vitality of the sperm.

In order to amplify the event, you must amplify yourself. Focus within and take the time to relax and feel connected. Rise in the morning to meditate and appreciate life, think good thoughts to feel happy, walk in nature, write poetry for your love, massage yourself, and massage your partner. The purpose of this is to increase your frequency to high level to increase the likelihood of bringing down a high soul. If you want your conception to be different than every other act, you have to show up differently and extend yourself beyond the usual. During the window of time, it is especially important to increase confidence in yourself, feel sexual, and expand your field in order to maintain, generate, and contain a powerful vitality. It should be a time of worship, where your house becomes the temple, you are the priestess, and he is the devotee.

During this window, you want to feel secure and develop an intimate conversation and connection with your partner. After your long bath, use almond oil to massage your body and then massage each other for the sake of pleasure, but don't partake in the act of intercourse until you know for sure you are ovulating. You want to build up to the event and connect in a different manner than you usually do. It is important that your minds are aligned and that mental frequency flows without any issues. In the days before conception, write or text each other frequently, flirt with your partner, and play together. Show him how confident you are in yourself and your sexuality. Make your bedroom into a temple by ensuring that it is clean and all the doors and windows are shut to create a closed and safe place for a high-energy encounter. While this is happening, you should also be in intimate mental contact with your baby and constantly letting the child and the Universe know that you are ready and willing to conceive.

DURING THE SEXUAL ENCOUNTER

When the seventy-two-hour window, is over make sure that your digestive system is empty and you have had a bowel movement. You don't want to have sex on a full stomach or when you are tired as it decreases your energy. Guru Jagat explained during *Creating the Aquarian Child Course* that in ancient yogic science there is a specific sequence to stimulate the erogenous zones and amplify the auric field before conscious conception. Before your sexual encounter, stimulate the following areas in this specific manner, for a minimum of thirty minutes, in order to amplify yourself and your partner.

Man to Woman:

Stimulate these erogenous zones in this order: Breasts from the outside inward, from the lower neck UP the spine, then lips, cheeks, ears, the spine, thighs inside to the outside, the calves, and finally the clitoris.

Woman to Man:

Stimulate these erogenous zones in this order: Massage the head and hair, then the lips, then top of the neck and down the spine (because they are often in their heads), roll the fascia around the spine (roll down smoothly), stop at the buttocks and massage, massage inside the thighs, then the testicles, and finally the penis. You can stimulate the penis and the heart region at the same time in order to connect the two centers; it could take months or even years to have these connected through this practice.

This can be done multiple times if necessary and with oil. The set can also be practiced the days leading up to the event. Think of it as an act of worshipping your partner and honoring the soul that you want to conceive. Or just consider it a relaxing massage, because that is what it is. Keep the breath strong and breathe in and out through an open O-shaped mouth to amplify your body sensations. During the sexual act you can also try breathing in synch, which is a little tricky but pleasurable as it increases energy. To do this place your lips together and open your mouth slightly while your partner breathes in and you breathe out and then vice versa, which essentially means you are breathing the same air together through your mouths and transferring your energy back and forth. During orgasm remember to breathe deeply. If you don't partake in any of the above, just remember this. Deep breath is essential for pleasurable sex. During your sacred encounter, speak to the baby and accept the soul into your body fully with conscious awareness.

When I conceived my second child, I knew it immediately and began to speak to her in my head by calling her down. Though I intuitively knew she was supposed to be born, we had just had our first baby, and it was a very stressful time. I panicked and bought the morning after pill within twenty-four hours, which was a pretty funny experience in itself. Imagine what it looks like walking up to the window of the pharmacy requesting this with a new baby in your arms. The pharmacist and I laughed out loud as if to say have you not learned your lesson yet. Needless to say, the pill did not work. When a soul wants to come down, it will without question. I witnessed many deliveries in the hospital where the women were religiously taking their birth control or had an IUD and still got pregnant. I have also seen women who had their tubes tied and others whose husbands have had a vasectomy become pregnant. These were extremely rare cases. Despite medical professionals deeming this impossible or caused by human error, it happens more than we know. The Universe is a powerful Creator.

TIME OF CONCEPTION

After orgasm leave the sperm inside as long as you can and meditate or pray after your encounter. Yogi Bhajan taught the sperm circles the egg exactly eight times and the force at which the sperm enters the egg creates the frequency of the child for the rest of their life. While remaining in a meditative state, when you are ready, you can sit up to just breathe in what might have happened. If you are sensitive, you will likely know if you have conceived. Do not urinate for a period of time (This is not the case if you are having regular sex not for conception.), and wash your face, ears, and feet with cold water. Cleanse your body and your teeth to honor yourself as a temple and allow for the new soul to come in. The act of conscious conception is like creating the holy trinity and the ultimate way for you to encounter Spirit in one of its most powerful and heart-opening acts. If you are conceiving through modern technology, you can still raise your energy before the act and maintain the connection to your partner and the child. Partake in the act of sex when you are ready and able in the same manner as above. Sex is not shameful; it is the art of pleasure and should be fully enjoyed on earth. Your choice to bring a child into this world in an aware manner is a holy act and complete rebellion against society's norms. With each conscious choice, you are helping to create a new earth and allowing the possibility of high-level souls to enter this plane of existence.

SAT KRIYA AS TAUGHT BY YOGI BHAJAN

This Kriya is a fundamental and simple meditation that you can do daily to increase your self-esteem and stimulate the sexual system. It is one of the best and most important meditations given by Yogi Bhajan because it works directly on stimulating the Kundalini energy and creating a high amount of energy in the system. It balances the lower chakras, increases the capacity of the heart, improves overall health, and balances sexual impulses.

Position: Sit on your heels and stretch the arms overhead so that elbows hug the ears. You can place a pillow behind your butt or under your feet and knees for comfort.

Mudra: Interlock the fingers except the first ones (index fingers), which point straight up. Men cross the right thumb over the left. Women cross the left thumb over the right.

Mantra: Begin to chant Sat Naam emphatically in a constant rhythm about eight times per ten seconds. Chant the sound Sat from the navel point and solar plexus, and pull the umbilicus all the way in and up, toward the spine. On Naam relax the belly.

Time: Lie down and relax flat on your back when you are done. You can do this between three to thirty-two minutes but not longer than sixty-two minutes.

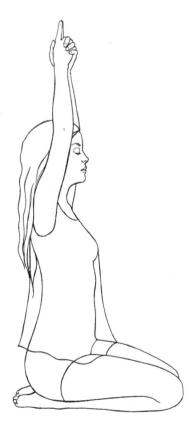

SECTION 2

SAFETY NEEDS DURING
PREGNANCY

"If the physiological needs are relatively well gratified, there then emerges a new set of needs, which we may categorize roughly as the safety needs (security, stability, dependency, protection, freedom from fear, anxiety, chaos, need for structure, order, law, and limits, strength in the protector and so on)…They may serve as the almost exclusive organizers of behavior, recruiting all the capacities of the organism in their service, and we may then fairly describe the whole organism as a safety- seeking mechanism… Some neurotic adults in our society are, in many ways, like unsafe children in their desire for safety. Their reactions are often to unknown psychological dangers in a world that is perceived to be hostile, overwhelming and threatening."

–ABRAHAM MASLOW

10. IMPROVING YOUR HEALTH DURING PREGNANCY

"Everything grows rounder and wider and weirder, and I sit here in the middle of it all and wonder who in the world you will turn out to be."

–CARRIE FISHER

The number one rule for maintaining a healthy diet during pregnancy is to focus on the types of foods you are eating and not attempt to replace nutrition through supplements. This means your diet should include plenty of fruits and vegetables, protein, grains, and lots of hydrating fluids. Some midwives will ask for a three-to-seven-day food diary, but not all doctors do this. I recommend that you record one whether your health professional asks or not and provide it to them for review. You may want to personally understand your long-term relationship with food and your own health status so that you are better prepared to eat the best foods for you and your baby. If money is an issue or you don't have time to prepare your food, make sure you plan and discuss these issues with your medical provider, family, and your boss.

During pregnancy, I highly suggest avoiding pesticides, antibiotics, and hormones because of the relative size of the fetus compared to the alarming concentration found in foods and products. If you can afford it, I would make it a priority to buy only organic foods whenever possible because of the higher nutritional value. If you choose to drink dairy, avoid products with bovine growth hormones; the packaging may have a label that reads "No rBGH." This is a concern in the United States but not in most European countries. Your meat and eggs should be free of antibiotics. Most fish and seafood have trace amounts of mercury, but ones that are particularly high include swordfish, mackerel, tuna, grouper, and halibut, so please avoid these. It is best to eat only wild caught fish if you can. Also monitor the facial and makeup products that you use, and try to buy to an organic brand. Other products to avoid while pregnant include junk food, caffeine, alcohol, drugs, food additives such as preservatives or coloring, raw or cured meats, and sushi. Avoid chocolate while you are pregnant as it is a stimulant and many brands are toxic

Throughout the day, make sure you drink at least two quarts water (preferably filtered) daily. This is especially important when it is hot outside. When I worked at a hospital in Los Angeles, one of the main reasons we saw patients in the triage room was because contractions started early as a result of dehydration in the summer months. While pregnant, make sure to eat at least eighty grams of protein daily, and if you are vegan, it is vital to take a vitamin B12 supplement. According to Elizabeth Davis, author of *Hearts & Hands: A Midwife's Guide to Pregnancy and Birth*, beyond a high-quality well-balanced diet, there are specific supplements that the pregnant woman should have. Proper nutrition and supplementation helps support babies in better brain and nervous system development and better sleep and behavioral patterns. The mother's health is also significantly increased, and there is a reduced chance of issues such as preeclampsia, postpartum depression, or preterm labor.

Aim to consume the following, preferably in your food:

√   **Vitamin E:** Sunflower seeds, almonds, hazelnuts, peanuts, spinach

√   **Folic Acid:** 400 - 800 mcg before and especially during the first twelve weeks of pregnancy. The dose is dependent upon previous conditions, so please seek medical advice. (brussels sprouts, eggs, broccoli, asparagus, brown rice)

√   **Vitamin C:** Papaya, broccoli, strawberries, bell peppers, brussels sprouts, cauliflower, cantaloupe, mustard greens, swiss chard, tomatoes

√   **Iron:** Pumpkin seeds, dried fruits, almonds

√   **Calcium:** Sesame butter and dark green leafy vegetables

√   **Magnesium:** Meat, fish, eggs, rice, and bread

√   **Zinc:** Spinach, pumpkin seeds, cashews, beef, chicken, kidney beans

√   **Omega-3 DHA and EPA:** Flaxseed oil or flaxseeds

Pregnant women should also maintain a regular exercise and relaxation program to assist them through the birth. The general rule for Western practitioners is to maintain the same level of exercise that you were doing before your pregnancy. The Kundalini Yogic Science recommends walking five miles a day until you give birth, which will help to balance weight and make your legs strong. In Japan, practitioners recommend five hundred squats per day for an easy labor. Daily vaginal toning or Kegels, before and after pregnancy, are also helpful to maintain pelvic floor muscles. Whatever you choose to do, just move and fit in time for relaxation or meditation. Completely let go at least once a day through dance or stretching. Start a form of relaxation the day you find out you are pregnant because it will help you through the birth significantly, and it will also help you to handle motherhood.

Emotional, intellectual, and social preparation for pregnancy and motherhood will be discussed throughout the book but are issues that need to be met starting before conception. Women need people to be able to vent to or communicate with especially during this time as a lot of issues may arise to be cleared. While you are pregnant, make a point to meet other pregnant women and create a concrete support group before you have your baby by joining community centers or classes. Intellectually prepare yourself by doing your own research, reading positive birth stories, and developing a simple birth and post birth plan.

EXERCISE:

When I was pregnant, my midwives gave me the recipe for a calcium-rich tea that I drank throughout pregnancy and while breastfeeding. Drinking it regularly can help to tone the uterus, increase energy, aid digestion, and calm the nervous system. The ingredients provide a lot of nutrients including calcium, magnesium, and iron. A large mug of the tea provides as much calcium as a cup of milk. If you cannot find these herbs locally, it is very easy to buy them in bulk online.

Red Raspberry Leaf: Has been used for centuries as a uterine tonic. It helps to normalize the uterus—increasing tone or relaxing the tissues if they become too irritable. Many midwives believe that it helps to shorten labor, decrease nausea, ease labor pains, and decrease the chance of excessive bleeding after birth. Some midwives only recommend using this herb and nettle in the second and third trimesters, so check with your provider.

Nettle: Highly nutritious and considered the best overall tonic. It affects the kidneys and helps to eliminate waste, while also increasing energy and the flow of breast milk.

Dandelion: A liver tonic, which increases bile flow helping you to break down fats. It helps with digestion and waste elimination. Nettle and dandelion are especially good at preventing edema.

Alfalfa: Contains vitamins A, D, E, and K. Vitamin K helps to reduce excessive bleeding after childbirth.

Rose Hips: A great source of Vitamin C.

Wild Oats, Lemon balm, Chamomile, and Lavender: Nourishing and calming to the nervous system.

Spearmint and Cinnamon: Tasty and add flavor! Mint is a great source of calcium and magnesium.

Stevia: Sugar substitute that is two hundred times sweeter than sugar with no calories! Only a small amount is needed.

To make the mixture: combine three or more of the herbs together. Make sure that you add one of the sweeter herbs for flavoring. When I make an infusion, I boil a large quart of water. I turn the boiling water off and let about a fistful of herbs (tucked into a tea filter sack) soak in the pot for four or more hours. I put the mixture in the fridge and drink it for the next few days like iced tea. Sometimes I'll add lemon, honey, carbonated water, or juice. Remember that with infusions, the longer the tea steeps, the more minerals and compounds are extracted. The tea keeps for up to three days in the refrigerator and four hours outside the fridge. You can also make small batches on the go: place one-half cup to two-thirds cup of herbal tea (in a tea ball or filter sack) in a glass jar of boiling water, cap it, and let it sit as long as thirty minutes to overnight in the fridge. Take it with you to work, or sip on it during your errands.

11. INCREASE YOUR COPING SKILLS IN PREGNANCY AND CHILDBIRTH

"A self-possessed woman in childbirth can be a powerful teacher for all (including herself) on the temporality, humility, and connectedness of life."

–ANI DIFRANCO

A woman's attitude and approach toward pregnancy, and life in general, tends to manifest during childbirth and the immediate time before. Women go through labor in a similar manner to the way they live, and because childbirth can be a hyped-up and emotional time, behaviors are often magnified. Coping skills are vital to have during this process, as certain personality characteristics and fears are potential risk factors for a high- or low-risk birth. Inner conflicts and anxieties that are not dealt with before labor can make a woman feel out of control, victimized, and in crisis. Some of these issues include physical or sexual abuse, self-image problems, dependency, passivity, resistance to change, and lack of support. If you have any of these problems, begin to address them before you give birth and preferably before you conceive. Women must become aware of their weaknesses and strengths so that they are capable of physically and psychologically enduring the labor process and becoming a mother. It is important to strengthen the support group, work through fears, integrate mind and body, and assume some inner control of life. This will help to create a healthy and safe foundation for yourself and the baby at birth.

HANDLING PAIN DURING LABOR AND SEXUAL ABUSE

When the average woman enters the delivery room, they have no idea of the extent of pain or discomfort they will feel, as every birth is different. Pain is a strange human experience, and perceptions vary a great deal. Reactions to pain are also different and are often influenced by the way individuals deal with stress or fear. As a labor and delivery nurse, I found that first-time moms often felt that the experience would never end. Some women entered the hospital and the first words they expressed were "I don't want to feel a thing." These women convinced themselves that they were not capable of giving birth naturally even before they knew what to expect because of programmed fear. Some were petrified, many felt unprepared, and others believed that labor was a complete inconvenience. No amount of education or discussion would change their mind, and early anesthesia or drugs were usually necessary and often detrimental to the labor progress.

Other women reacted to labor pain as if they were being wounded or physically hurt. In these cases, many of the women had a history of sexual abuse that they had not dealt with. Instead of relaxing into the contractions, and focusing on opening the pelvis, they resisted, sometimes taking on the patterned condition of the victim. One of the first and most important questions I asked my patients was whether they had a history or rape or sexual abuse, because it is likely that one out of three women has. This is vital to know because it can energetically impede the opening of the cervix or relaxation of the pelvis. In my experience, sexually abused women blocked connection to their second chakra, or their womb, out of fear. In one specific case, I had a patient who began to remember and react to past sexual abuse she had forgotten about, or buried in her subconscious, during labor. She became triggered and inconsolable, which ended with a traumatic C-section for the mother and baby. If you have a history of physical or sexual abuse, please seek counsel before your birth in order to better prepare yourself for motherhood.

A NEED TO CONTROL LEADS TO SURRENDER OR RESISTANCE

It was also common for mothers to enter the hospital with a list of items that they wanted to refuse during pregnancy: no IVs, no monitors, no students, particular room requests, and no interventions. These women were usually intense, Type A, often high powered, and older. Sometimes their birth plans were ten to twelve pages long and detailed. This was always a big indicator of a patient that would likely become incredibly fearful or distrusting and thus end up with more interventions then the average patient. When fear is increased during childbirth, the cervix will not open, which leads to a higher rate of medical or surgical intervention. Control is a survival mechanism and the need for it often leads to a great deal of internal stress. Most hospitals want every mother to feel safe and agree with as many requests as possible under the right circumstances. However, if you do not want any of the interventions that the hospital is going to offer you, I highly recommend not delivering at a medical center if that is an option for you. If you are an individual who thrives on controlling your environment, you may think you will feel safer in a hospital, but this is not always the case for the super Type A personality

All women should have the option to choose what you want, but you are likely not going to get most of those choices met in the environment of the average medical center. The longer list of items a woman attempts to control, the higher tendency there is for intervention, especially during a hospital delivery. Birth cannot always be managed from an intellectual standpoint. It is a mind-body connection, and the more you separate the mind from the body, the more likely it is that medical staff will insist on helping. If you desire to write a birth plan, be prepared and know your options. Also know that you are entering a hospital, and many of these facilities are focused on business and protocol. They are there to help you birth your baby in the best way they see fit. If you feel that the medical team is moving too fast, ask them to slow down and explain what is going on and offer options. Trust your intuition. Make sure you understand how the medical center works before you show up in labor especially if you are working with a group of doctors on call or if you are not sure when your chosen health provider will arrive. If you are delivering in a teaching hospital with a large staff and you are faced with making decisions with a younger doctor or a student, always ask for the chief resident, charge nurse, or chief doctor to come in and speak with you. Hospitals like to keep control, and that is why they maintain a list of interventions during birth. If you are interested in reducing the amount of interventions, consider using a midwife, birth center, or having a homebirth instead if your health condition allows.

Know Thyself

Understand the basic principle that things do not always go as planned and it is necessary to have adequate coping skills. You must get to know yourself; your attitude toward life and the way you deal with problems will come up during labor and especially into motherhood. Here are some questions that all women should ask themselves as they prepare for labor and delivery. The following qualities tend to lead to a low-risk childbirth. If you are pregnant and have any issues in the following areas (Which we all do!), start to address them now so that you will be prepared during birth. If you have already had your baby, these are still good questions as they affect the way you parent. Answer these questions and then begin to locate areas in your life that you could grow or need to heal.

EXERCISE:

✓ Do you consider yourself an active and independent woman? Do you like to take charge or sit back and watch others? Can you find a balance here?

✓ Are you able to take support from others? If someone tries to help you, how do you react?

✓ Are you able to deal with changes in an appropriate manner, or do you tend to resist? Do you resist people, places, changes, or yourself?

✓ Is there anything you are scared of? If so, are these fears being worked through?

✓ Do you think of yourself as a sexual being, with a healthy attitude toward sexuality and your capabilities as a woman? (I do not mean a sexual object.) Are you comfortable connecting to your reproductive organs, relaxing your pelvis, and focusing on your cervix?

✓ Are you clear and honest in your communication? Do you tend to lie to yourself or others? If so, when and why does this happen?

✓ Do your spiritual beliefs match your ideal pregnancy and birth? What is your ideal birth? What does it look like? Begin to create this daily in your mind through visualization and positive feelings or projection.

✓ Have you been physically or sexually abused? If so, have you dealt with these issues? (Women who have experienced sexual abuse are more likely to have dysfunctional or high-risk labors.)

✓ Do you ever consider yourself powerless? If so, what types of situations does this happen in, and how do you deal?

✓ Do you and your partner have a loving relationship? Do you trust one another? Who in your life have you not trusted and why?

✓ Does your partner ever speak over you or speak for you? Is your voice and opinion heard?

I AM A WOMAN AFFIRMATION PRACTICE AS TAUGHT BY YOGI BHAJAN

"These are the strongest affirmations you can ever utter. The moment you make the tongue rotate, watch the tip of the upper palate stimulate your entire psyche and force the neurons to adjust their balance right there on the spot. The hypothalamus immediately communicates with the subconscious memory to release your strength and all the strength of every woman grand, grand, great, great, great, super—two million generations from which your egg has come through, and confront the spermatozoa…

God Made Me a Woman. The infinity. Woman contains the man in it. God is responsible for making it. You do not take the blame. This gets rid of the blame. You recognize your ego to be God's Will. Nobody can get rid of ego, but you can convert your ego into God's Will. I Am a Woman to Be This is an affirmation of your own honour, nobility, self-love, creativity, to get rid of the crisis and conflict that are within you. Now Now Now It is the elevating power to face the now. Capture and elevate yourself above time. You say three times: In the past I have done it. I am going to do it. I am going to do it no matter what. "–Yogi Bhajan

Sit comfortably and recite these affirmations. Time: Three to eleven minutes. You can also write this down or just write "I am a Woman" over and over to remember your power.

God Made Me a Woman, I Am a Woman to Be, Now, Now, Now

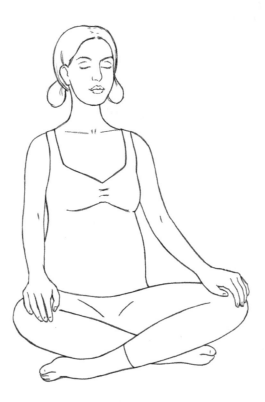

"I did it!" The Birth of Levi Samuel
– April's Birth Story

To help give some context to Levi's birth story and what it meant to me, it helps to understand a little about my experience with my first birth. With Lily's pregnancy, we didn't think much about picking a care provider, and just went with the first recommendation we got from the fertility specialist we had been seeing (we did not require any treatments to get pregnant with her, but after 21 months of trying, we had started some testing when we finally got pregnant!). The doctor seemed nice enough, we really liked the hospital he was at, and it was directly across the street from Myles' fire station at the time. The office was nice, and they did ultrasounds often, right there in the office. I was interested in a natural birth, but having never experienced labor before, I decided to go in with an open mind and basically just see how far I could make it without drugs. I thought I was comfortable with the idea of an epidural if I felt like I needed it, although the reality was that I was just scared of the unknown! Deep down, I really didn't want the added risks to myself or the baby, and I hated the thought of a needle in my spine.

I went to all of my appointments, where I spent 30 or more minutes in the waiting room, and all of about 5 minutes with the doctor each time. By the time I hit 39 weeks, he was already trying to schedule my induction. Knowing an average healthy pregnancy can last 42 weeks or more, I wasn't comfortable with this. I was able to push for a few extra days, and an induction was scheduled for the day before I hit 41 weeks. I prayed I would start labor on my own, and thankfully I did, 3 days after my due date. While in labor I was stuck to the monitors, which kept me from moving around like I had hoped to do. I had a room FULL of people. These were people I love dearly, but being a very introverted person who hates being the center of attention, it hindered my ability to relax and focus on getting through the contractions. One of the nurses kept repeatedly asking me if/when I wanted my epidural and finally, around 6-7cm dilated, I gave in and said yes. I wasn't to the point that I couldn't handle the pain, but at that point with everything happening the way it was, I didn't believe in myself to make it all the way through without it.

Lily was born healthy, caught by her daddy, but she had inhaled meconium in the womb and so I didn't get to hold her right away. I sadly, didn't get that moment of instantly falling in love with your baby (in fact, I felt like it took several weeks to get to that point). I watched while they scooped her up and suctioned her lungs and very, very roughly handled her...flipping her all around and rubbing her down/wiping her off. They cut her cord right away, even though I had wanted to do delayed cord clamping. I asked to nurse her, as I had hoped to right away, and was told I couldn't because of the meconium. I had to push to even get the skin to skin time I had so looked forward to. I was then given pitocin without my knowledge, which I had specifically asked NOT to receive and was stitched up, as I had a small tear (that I believe was mainly due to not being able to feel anything for the pushing stage). As I finally nursed Lily for the first time, the pushy epidural nurse who had also been so rough with my sweet baby, made it a point to tell me that it had been more than 20 minutes and my baby wasn't getting anything at that point and that I didn't need to let her use me as a pacifier (all horribly incorrect information that can be detrimental to a nursing relationship).

Breastfeeding got off to a rocky start and I was quickly cracked and bleeding and in pain, despite being told by a lactation nurse that Lily's latch was fine. Due to not having a good latch, I believe Lily wasn't transferring the milk effectively, and therefore nursed vigorously and almost constantly which just led to more pain and damage to me. Between that and nurses checking mine and baby's vitals every couple of hours, I got no sleep at all. By the time I got home, I was exhausted, in pain, and doubting my abilities as a mom. I felt very down for the first couple of months and believe that I suffered from slight post partum depression. After this experience, I knew I wanted better for my next baby.

When we found out we were expecting again, I had already decided I wanted to see a midwife instead of an OB/gyn as long as the baby and I were healthy and the pregnancy low risk. I had learned about a very local midwife, Jennie Joseph, and her birth center from a couple of other moms in the area, and called and got set up right away. When I had concerns about low hormone levels in the beginning of the pregnancy, Jennie allowed me to come in earlier than usual to have bloodwork done and check on everything. Baby and I were healthy throughout the pregnancy, and I looked forward to every appointment at The Birth Place. Wait times were short, and I never once felt rushed. Whether I saw Jennie or one of the other staff, I always left with every question answered and a smile on my face. Most importantly, I felt like my wishes for the pregnancy and birth were important to them. I wasn't just stuck with whatever "hospital protocol" happened to be. It was my body, my baby, my birth and I felt like I was in charge of making the decisions, with knowledgeable support to back me up. That kind of respect was very empowering!

As my due date approached, I prepared myself by reading other women's birth stories, reading books like Ina May's Guide to Childbirth, and lots of prayer and positive affirmations. I reminded myself often that I am fearfully and wonderfully made and that my body was created for this. I thought of Mary giving birth to Jesus in a stable and all the other women who had come before me who had given birth safely to their babies. I told myself "You can do this" and reminded myself that birth is not a sickness or a disease or an emergency. Birth is a normal (albeit intense) bodily function that I don't have to be afraid of. God has not given me a spirit of fear, but of power and love and a sound mind. Positive thinking played a big role in preparing for Levi's arrival.

On my due date, January 21st, I decided to lay down for a nap with Lily. Around 4:30pm I woke up because I felt a "pop." When I opened my eyes, I wasn't sure if I had dreamt the sensation or not. But as I went to roll over to climb out of the bed, I felt several huge gushes of water that left no doubt in my mind (thank God for having a waterproof pad down on the bed!). I was immediately excited and shaky and nervous all at the same time. I knew that if I had been seeing an OB and delivering at a hospital, they would want me to come in right away. If labor had not started within 12 hours I would likely have been started on pitocin, which causes harder contractions and more stress on the baby, which increases the chance I would need an epidural, which would increase my risk of a c-section (look up "cascade of interventions"). Thankfully I knew that being allowed to labor at home, without anyone doing unnecessary vaginal exams, free to move around as I pleased, meant that my risk of infection was low.

I called the birth center and quickly got a call back from Jennie. I told her that my water had broken but I wasn't feeling any contractions yet. She told me not to worry and to just call her before I went to bed if there still wasn't anything happening. She would have me come in the morning to evaluate. I was able to eat and relax, and was so grateful for such a low stress experience. I was starving and had a small meal every couple of hours. Scrambled eggs with spinach and feta cheese, a banana, ¼ of a turkey and ham sub, 3 or 4 handfuls of almonds, a big green smoothie, a bowl of lentil soup. My body obviously knew I was getting ready to work hard. I would have been restricted to clear fluids and ice chips at this point had I been in a hospital. I showered and finished up last minute preparations for the baby, bounced on my birth ball and watched tv.

I had sporadic contractions starting in the evening. I tried to time them but they were very inconsistent and while growing in intensity, they were still mostly mild…10 minutes, 7 minutes, 12 minutes, 5 minutes, 12 more minutes. They eventually started to get stronger, averaging about 7 minutes apart. When I finally decided I should try to lay down and rest, my contractions stopped for a couple of hours. As much as this made me nervous that labor may not progress on its own, in hindsight, I believe my body was just allowing me to rest when I needed it. By the next morning I was ready to help move things along. I sniffed my clary sage oil and bounced on my birth ball. I texted Jennie with an update, and let her know my labor had pretty much stopped. Her reply was something that became another positive affirmation that I repeated to myself for the rest of my labor. She told me not to push myself too hard. She said, "Baby will come." I immediately let go of the pressure I was putting on myself to make something happen. And while I wanted to continue to gently, naturally encourage my labor to progress, I was no longer stressed about it. Baby will come.

The next thing on my list to try to get things going, I was embarrassed to try, and honestly am a little embarrassed to share. But it was EXTREMELY effective to start contractions, is totally natural with no side effects and could save someone else from unnecessary interventions…so I will! Nipple stimulation (with your hands, breast pump, shower, whatever). Anyone who has nursed a baby for any length of time knows the science behind this. After birth, the baby's suckling causes contractions that help the uterus shrink back down to size (also known as afterpains...ouuuuch). It took all of 10 minutes to trigger contractions that were pretty intense and hitting every 3-5 minutes. This continued for the next hour and 15 minutes when Jennie asked me to come in. We got there around noon, when I was checked and told I was already 6cm dilated. The contractions were intense enough at this point that when one would hit I would have to close my eyes and focus on breathing through them. I found that I needed to be standing and bracing myself on a wall when they hit. Myles was always right there to apply pressure to my lower back, as my labor was almost completely felt in my back. In between contractions, I was comfortable, having conversations, unpacking our bag in the room we had chosen (light, white and blue bedding, lots of sunlight pouring in, very cheery).

Once I knew we were staying, the contractions came on faster and stronger. I never reached a point where I thought I couldn't do it, because I had so ingrained it in my mind that I could. But I definitely reached a point where I didn't want to do it anymore. I kept telling myself that I WAS doing it. That I couldn't run away from it, so I needed to surrender to it. I wanted to be in the water, because I knew it would help me relax, but I didn't want it to slow things down so I waited (had I known how close I was, I wouldn't have worried about this). I finally got to the point that it felt like the contractions weren't stopping. There was little break in between them and any movement I made seemed to trigger another one. I asked Jennie to fill up the pool and couldn't wait to get in, but it felt like a marathon just to move myself the few feet across the room to get to it.

Climbing in the warm water was heavenly. The pain of the contractions stayed the same, but I felt every other muscle in my body relax, which really helped me to cope with the pain. I felt most comfortable on my hands and knees, and Myles got into whatever uncomfortable position he needed to be able to keep applying counter-pressure to my back (I seriously could NOT have done this without him, he was amazing!). When I started to feel my body pushing, I thought I was doing something wrong. I was convinced that there was no way I was THAT close to having a baby. Jennie was amazing at this point. While I didn't make much noise, as I was totally in the zone, she knew when I was close. She knew when I was getting "pushy" just by watching and listening to me. She knew just what I needed to hear. When she started to tell me to "focus on your bottom" I knew it was ok to let myself push a little. It was about this time when another contraction hit and I involuntarily pushed a lot! I decided to go with it and focus on bringing my baby down. Pushing was AMAZING. Every bit of pain from the contractions disappeared when I was pushing. And while it was a very intense sensation, once I surrendered to it, and really felt the amount of power coming from my body behind those pushes, I felt amazingly strong. Jennie checked me at this point and told me I still had just a little bit of cervix in the way. She checked on the baby with the doppler, and told me that she wanted to get me up into a squat for the next contraction. The LAST thing I wanted to do was move at that point, but I trusted her so I did.

As soon as my feet hit the bottom of the pool, the next contraction hit and I was pushing as hard as I could, with Jennie's encouragement the whole time. In that one push, I felt intense pressure, and then relief as the head came out. I never felt the "ring of fire" you hear about, or any other pain at this point…just pressure and then relief (no tears whatsoever). I leaned back against the side of the pool, reached down, and could feel my baby's hair and even his facial features. Myles told me after the fact that as soon as he saw Levi's face, he was sure it was a boy. My joy quickly turned to a moment of slight panic as I realized I still had to deliver the shoulders and body…I had forgotten about that part in the moment, and assumed it would be difficult. Jennie asked me to grab my knees on the next contraction and with one last quick push, Levi was out of the water and on my chest, again with no pain. All I could think was "I can't believe I just did that!" Myles laughed as he announced it was a boy (I forgot to even look), and I held him up just to make sure. I was ecstatic. I couldn't believe how perfect, and calm and alert he was. Jennie immediately grabbed her phone and started snapping pictures for us, and I am so very grateful she was able to capture those moments.

We moved to the bed to deliver the placenta, and I nursed my baby boy for the first time. I was on such a natural high (oxytocin rocks!). I kept looking at him, smiling and saying, "Hi baby! We did it!" as he stared back at me. I asked him what his name was, and Myles and I agreed right away that he was a "Levi". He stayed on my chest for at least an hour with his cord and placenta still attached. The cord continued to pulse for that entire hour, pumping all of Levi's blood back into his little body. When it finally stopped pulsing, Myles cut the cord. We were asked if we wanted the vitamin K shot or the antibiotic eye ointment, both of which we declined and no questions were asked. We finally weighed the baby, and they did a newborn exam right on the bed with us. I was able to shower, get a snack, introduce Lily to her brother, and we were all able to just enjoy each other for a few hours. After going over some simple instructions for what to do in the next few days, they checked on baby and I one last time and only 6 hours after Levi was born, we were able to take him home. We have been in babymoon bliss ever since!

This birth was empowering, and I feel very blessed for the privilege I had to experience it. It has caused me to grow spiritually, to fall more deeply in love with my husband and also my daughter who makes me proud every day with the love she shows for her baby brother. It has boosted my confidence in my abilities as a mother. It has removed any self-doubt and given me a new appreciation for my body and what it is capable of. But most of all, it has made me realize that, with God's help, I can accomplish anything I set my mind to.

12. SUPPORT DURING CHILDBIRTH

"If a doula effect were a drug, it would be considered unethical
not to use it."

–KENNELL

Doulas provide continuous emotional and physical support during labor, and they are an amazing addition to increase the wellbeing of the mother throughout birth. Using a doula during childbirth will significantly improve the health of the mother and baby and ultimately increase safety. Many individuals are afraid to have someone they don't really know that well in their birth room. This is completely understandable. Honestly, there are some doulas that are not meant for the job—just as there are medical professionals not meant for theirs. In my opinion, the best doulas are the ones who work with your nurse, midwife, or doctor and have an intuitive presence. Doulas are not medically trained and should not make medical decisions for you. They also should not speak for you during labor. They are there to provide support through massage, imagery, and guidance of body positions.

Women need a continuous presence during childbirth, and in a medical setting, it is very difficult to get this. At some birthing centers, nurses are given two to three active laboring women. There is no way that they can be in each room for extended periods, and these mothers are left alone to figure out how to manage on their own. Many nurses prefer that their patients get an epidural because taking care of a natural laboring woman is not in their comfort zone and is often too physically and psychologically challenging. Nurses are not trained to be doulas, just as doulas are not trained to be nurses. Each person has a separate but important role in birth. If you are lucky enough to have one that is both thank your stars.

It is difficult to research how deep the human need for caring and nurturing is, but during labor it is a priority. If this is your first baby, or even if it is your third baby, looking into getting a doula could be incredibly beneficial. No amount of education, or even support from your partner, can prepare you for birth, and mothers often feel alone in the process. Having a woman next to you continuously to make you feel safe could significantly change your experience. Dr. Marshall Klaus, M.D. and Dr. John Kennell, M.D. have done a substantial amount of research on doulas and helped to start an international organization to train doulas worldwide called DONA. Here are some of their findings:

✓ For first-time mothers, the presence of a doula shortened labor by an average of two hours and reduced the rate of cesarean section by fifty percent.

✓ Doula support could save the healthcare system an average of two billion dollars per year by reducing epidurals, fevers, surgery, and interventions.

✓ A doula reduces the need for anesthesia by her continuous presence

Doulas are one of the most effective ways to improve labor and delivery outcomes and increase safety because of their continuous presence and support. The cost for a doula ranges from five hundred dollars to fifteen hundred dollars depending on the area where you live and the level of experience. Personally, I had doulas at both of my births and couldn't have done it any other way. During my first birth, my doula saved the day when she called the midwife to come in a rush. At the time I wasn't thinking straight as my birth progressed fast and I could not believe that I was in active labor. When she saw me, she immediately called my midwife who greeted me at the door when I was at eight centimeters and feeling ready to push. I chose to have both my babies at home, and the doulas I hired helped with organization, support, timing of midwife arrival, and pain control through their presence. I recommend that first-time mothers choose more experienced doulas. Most doulas include prenatal and postpartum visits with their cost. If you plan to have an epidural at your birth, and you are absolutely set on your choice, a doula may not be the right choice for you. I found that when my patients received an epidural, the doula's support was no longer needed in most cases, because the mother needed the time to rest. If you are on the edge about whether you want an epidural, a doula may be the person who can help you ride that wave and take you across the threshold. With more human support, you will be less likely to receive interventions.

EXERCISE:

SOME QUESTIONS OR CONCERNS TO CONSIDER WHEN HIRING A DOULA:

- ✓ How many births has she attended? (Note even inexperienced doulas could be incredibly helpful as it is often natural intuition and a mothering presence that is needed.)

- ✓ Has she had children herself?

- ✓ Have her provide you with birth stories of other clients.

- ✓ Is she available after the birth, and how long does she stay to support new mothers?

- ✓ Does she have experience with breastfeeding support?

✓ How does she feel about interventions at the hospital?

✓ What are her communication skills like, and how does she support women through birth? Does she use touch, language, or massage?

✓ Does she have a working relationship with the hospital or birthing center? How does she deal with adversity or change?

✓ Does she advocate for her patients, and how does she prefer to communicate with the medical team?

✓ What is her background in and how does this support your birth? Ask for references from other clients.

✓ Make sure to meet with her to ensure that she understands the labor process and approaches your decisions in a nonjudgmental way.

13. ELECTRONIC FETAL MONITORING AND SAFETY

"I believe that it is beneficial to monitor a baby's heart rate during labor. But the majority of … women receive the wrong type of fetal monitoring for their situation. They receive something called continuous electronic monitoring instead of intermittent auscultation."

–REBECCA DEKKER, PHD, RN, APRN

The electronic fetal monitor (EFM) was enthusiastically introduced into the medical system during the 1960s and took off in the 1980s in hopes that continuously detecting the baby's heart rate would ensure safety and lower the risk of perinatal death. EFM is a method for examining the condition of a baby in the uterus by noting any unusual changes in the baby's heart rate. It is performed late in pregnancy or during labor and can be utilized either externally or internally in the womb. External EFM involves placing electrodes on the mother's belly, which measure fetal heartbeat and strength of contractions. Internal EFM can only be done once the mother's cervix is partially dilated and involves an electrode being placed into the uterus and attached to the baby's scalp.

Ina May Gaskin, author of *Birth Matters: A Midwife's Manifesta*, explained that when the EFM was introduced it increased the rate of cesarean section because doctors had not expected that "the lowered fetal heart rates during uterine contractions that could be picked up for the first time with the continuous monitor… were absolutely normal." Many heart rate tracings are identified as abnormal when the baby is not in distress. Continuous EFM is highly sensitive and has the ability to identify fetuses that are distressed, but it also has low specificity, or the ability to identify those that are not in distress. The EFM therefore has a high false positive rate, meaning the machine can be wrong and detrimental in some cases.

Walsh described a systematic review involving twelve studies and thirty-seven thousand women comparing continuous EFM to intermittent auscultation (listening by hand with a fetoscope periodically after a contraction) and found that there were no differences between the two in perinatal death rates, Apgar scores (test to assess health of newborn), infant intensive care admissions, or cerebral hypoxia (lack of oxygen to the brain). EFM halved neonatal seizures but also resulted in a significant increase in cesarean sections and assisted vaginal births with the use of instruments such as forceps and more recently vacuums. Ina May Gaskin explained, "The techno-medical model of maternity care, unlike the midwifery model, is comparatively new on the world scene, having existed for barely two centuries. This male-derived framework for care is a product of the industrial revolution…Pregnancy and labor are seen as illnesses, which, in order not to be harmful to mother or baby, must be treated with drugs and medical equipment. Within the techno-medical model of birth, some medical intervention is considered necessary for every birth, and birth is safe only in retrospect." Electronic monitoring is usually used because Pitocin, a drug that alters labor and increases contractions, is started. Or before this, the woman is given a drug to soften and open the cervix. Interventions lead to more interventions and with that the natural aspect of birth is disregarded. For many women, this can lead to loss of control and series of unplanned birth events that may cause stress of fear.

The United States Preventive Services Task Force states that the EFM is not recommended in low-risk women and that there is insufficient evidence regarding its use in high-risk women despite recognizing that many hospitals use EFM as common, non-evidence-based practice. Evidence shows that intermittent listening with a fetoscope is just as reliable as EFM, and in most cases takes away much of the fear involved in birth, resulting in fewer cesareans. So why is this method still in practice? This is because continuously monitoring a woman in labor requires less human contact. It is also needed because of the increased use of synthetic drugs to enhance or start labor, which makes birth more unpredictable because of the possibility of distress of the baby.

Generally, one nurse can "monitor" several patients at a time from a local station. When your nurse is not in your room, she is watching your baby in another one. Doctors can monitor an entire unit from one office. This in turn lowers costs and shows evidence, via the long strands of paper, that the baby was watched throughout labor if a courtroom was ever involved. Technology has a way of creating the illusion that we are progressing. This is not always the case, and there is data to prove it. Hospital staff and even parents tend to depend on these machines, creating a mind-body split. Sometimes the monitor becomes more important than the internal experience. Don't let this happen to you. Remain empowered and always ask questions. If you can, try hard to not pay attention to the machine in order to reduce your fears and stay safe in the labor room. I have seen many parents become emotionally drawn in by a computer and the sound of the heartbeat in the room, rather than focus on what the body and baby are doing inside. The mother is in labor not the machine. Feel the connection to your baby internally not externally.

If you cannot have intermittent monitoring at the location you deliver, ask the nurse to move the machine out of your line of vision. Maybe she can even cover it with a blanket so it is her concern and not yours. Ask her to turn down the noise and assess how you can best move around the room. The ancient ways of birthing through continuous human contact are still relevant and vital to health and safety for mothers and newborns.

THE DIVINE SHIELD MEDITATION FOR PROTECTION AND POSITIVITY AS TAUGHT BY YOGI BHAJAN

"It is difficult to focus on your higher feelings and sensitivity if you feel fearful and unprotected. If the universe seems hostile, uncaring and non-responsive it is easy to become filled with cynicism, despair and hopelessness. In that depressed state it is impossible to sense the fullness and possibilities of Life. It is very difficult to solve the very problems that upset you. The sound of "ma" calls on compassion and protection. It is the same sound that a baby uses to call on the mother. In this case, your soul is the child and the universe becomes the mother. If you call, she will come to your aid and comfort. When this shield is strong, it is easy to sense the tide of the universe, the Tao. You become spontaneous and vital as you move in rhythm with the greater Reality of which you are part. When the shield is strong you are protected from the impact of your own past actions. You are like a great ship that turns toward God and Reality and then must cross the waves of your own wake that you created by your past actions. The shield keeps you alert and awake to the real task of your life."

–KUNDALINI RESEARCH INSTITUTE

Eyes: Closed and focused at the brow point.

Posture and Mudra: Raise the right knee up with the right foot flat on the ground, toes pointing straight ahead. Place the sole of the left foot against the arch and ankle of the right foot. The ball of the left foot rests just in front of the ankle bone of the right foot.

Make a fist of the left hand, and place it on the ground beside the hip. Use this to balance the posture. Bend the right elbow, and place it on the top of the right knee. Bring the right hand back along the side of the head with the palm facing the ear. Form a shallow cup of the right palm. Then bring it against the skull so that it contacts the skull below the ear but stays open above the ear. It is as if you formed a cup of the hand to amplify a faint sound that you want to hear.

Mantra: Inhale deeply and chant Maaa in a long, full, smooth sound. Project the sound as if someone is listening to you. As you chant, listen to the sound current, and let it vibrate your body.

Time: Continue for eleven to thirty-one minutes. Then change the legs and hands to the other side. Continue for an equal amount of time. Start slowly. Learn to hold the concentration into the sound.

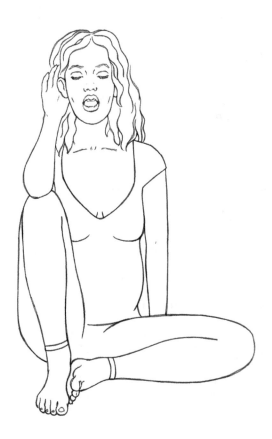

Choosing a Home Birth
– Erin's Birth Story

I don't know how it happened or when it happened, but sometime after moving to Victoria BC I became an earthy-granola mom. It happened before I was even pregnant, before I had ever thought about having a kid—but it happened.

Victoria is on Vancouver Island, just a short ferry ride away from Vancouver. Folks in this town are laid back, casual and very into their health food, yoga, community gardens, micro-breweries and Birkenstocks. When I first moved to Victoria from my yuppy life in Vancouver I hated it. Now I am guilty on all accounts. So I guess it shouldn't come as a surprise that when I found out I was pregnant, I started to consider a home birth. Over Christmas this year, my sister-in-law asked me why I wanted a home birth, and I muttered something about wanting to avoid interventions at the hospital (which is true, our local hospital has a 35% C-section rate), but when I came home and thought about it some more, I realized that I didn't really choose a home birth. Much like my accidental immersion into the Victoria lifestyle, it chose me.

I'M SO GLAD I DID IT

Around month 4, after the horrible nausea and vomiting had subsided, I recall discussing the possibility of a home birth with my midwives Jody and Astrid. At that time I thought it was an interesting idea but didn't seriously consider it. But sometime later in my pregnancy, as I started to really bond with our baby, the idea of having the birth at home really started to appeal to me. I started researching with fervour. I read Ina May Gaskin's books. I watched the Business of Being Born, I quizzed my doula and midwives and scoured the internet for information on birth pools. By the time I was 37 weeks and we could officially plan for a home birth I was sure that was the way to go. We were in.

THE BIRTH DAY

My husband likes to joke that, apart from the fact that we had a baby on September 16, it started and ended like any other day. That morning, my husband, Adam, had dropped me off at the dog park around 7 am for a morning walk and headed off to work. I walked along the ocean for about an hour and sat down for a while to take in the amazing view of the Olympic peninsula across the water. We were having a gorgeous fall and, already on maternity leave, I was determined to enjoy every day before baby came. I had one last file to drop off at the office that morning so I went in around 10:30 and discussed the file with my colleague who was covering for me. I felt some contractions, but they felt like braxton hicks so I didn't think anything of it. By the time I was at home around 11:00, things were very different.

I called Adam at work and told him I wasn't SURE but it felt like I might be having labour contractions. Adam said he'd be home by lunch - I told him to take his time. This could be false labour and, if it wasn't, we'd probably be at this for a nice long while anyway. I called our doula and midwives, everyone said they'd check in a little while later and I started to get the ingredients together for chilli. This was going to be my birth project; something to keep my mind off of the contractions.

I wasn't due until September 21 and was certain I would be overdue. After all, this was my first baby. I had spent the past three months psyching myself up for a long labour a week or so after I was due. Baby had other plans. About twenty minutes after I'd made my calls, my contractions got really intense. A woman from the diaper service stopped by to drop off our cloth diapers. We chatted for a bit and another contraction hit me. Doubled over, I laughed and said that labour had started so her timing couldn't be better. She asked whether my water broke and before she could finish her sentence, as if on cue, I felt a gush of water between my legs.

After my water broke labour seemed to go into hyperdrive. By the time Adam made it home at 12:15 my contractions were about five minutes apart. I couldn't stand up on my own any more during the contractions. We decided to head to the shower. While I was in the shower, our doula, Corrine, arrived and Adam called the midwife to update her. She was on her way.

My contractions continued to get stronger and stronger and Adam and Corrine took turns between helping me in the shower and scrambling to try and set up our birth pool and to prepare our bedroom. I couldn't understand how anyone could possibly do a birth project in labour. This was way too intense! Then I had a horrible realization. There was no way I was going to make it through this process without an epidural. The contractions were like nothing I'd ever felt before and I just didn't think I could do it. I cursed all the hippy-dippy granola moms whose stories I'd read months before about "rushes" and feeling love for their baby and feeling at peace. That was all crap. Crap crap crap. If this was how I was going to feel for the next 12 hours I was going to need drugs.

When my midwife, Astrid, arrived between 1:30 and 2:00, I willed myself out of the shower for her to check my cervix. I was stunned when she proclaimed "8 cm! Good work mama!" Knowing that I only had a couple of cm left to go renewed my determination to have this baby at home and without drugs. Now that I knew this wasn't the early labour pains I'd been told I'd have for 6 hours, I knew I could do this.

At that point, it was pretty clear we were not going to have time to fill up that birth pool. Jody, our other midwife, cancelled her last couple of appointments and hopped in a cab to come be the second midwife at our birth. This baby was wasting no time.

A couple of hours blurred by. I laboured leaning against a birth ball, on Adam, on Corrine, on the toilet - I was willing to try anything to get through the contractions at this point. Adam and Corrine plied me with juice and honey in between contractions to keep my energy up. Apparently I asked twice to go to the hospital for drugs but I don't remember that at all. I do remember my husband reminding me to "let my monkey do it" - a reminder to let go of my thoughts and anxieties and trust that my body would be able to figure this all out.

After about two hours of intense contractions coming two minutes apart or so (with 30 second breaks in between) I was finally ready to push. It's funny, when you see labor depicted in the movies, it always seems that the actual birth of the baby, the pushing, is the most painful part. It wasn't like that for me. I was DELIGHTED to finally get to push. Finally all this pain was for something. We were going to meet our little one so soon!

We moved from the living room to the bedroom. I began trying to push and my midwives cheered me on as we made progress with each contraction. In between contractions I had about two minutes of rest. Those two moments were incredible and I was able to take the shortest of naps (seriously - at this point I was exhausted and two minutes of sleep was AWESOME) or we chatted about how to get through the next contraction, what position to try. This is the time that I will always remember when I reflect on my birth. Everyone was calm. Baby was calm and happy. We were at home, in our bed and the sun was streaming in through the window.

After about 30 minutes, Astrid suggested I try pushing in a squat position for the next contraction. Jody handed me a mirror so I could see the progress we were making and I started to laugh as I saw the baby's head for the first time. We were SO close. I went back to my side and Astrid asked me NOT to push for the next few contractions so she could make sure I wouldn't tear and to check the position of the umbilical cord. After pushing for so long NOT pushing was even harder. Adam was a rock star the whole time supporting my leg as I pushed. After a couple more pushes the baby's head emerged. One more push and the rest of the body slid out.

Astrid caught the baby and then asked me to reach down and grab my baby. For a split second I didn't understand what she was saying. Reach down and grab my baby? I have a baby? And what? Why wasn't she wrapping him before she gave him to me. Adam nudged me and I launched into action. I pulled the baby onto my chest and Astrid quickly covered us both with blankets. We snuggled in, Adam, the baby and I, and I laugh-cried. The baby was so tiny, and so perfect.

Astrid and Jody asked me if I wanted to know if it was a boy or a girl. We were so excited that we had ANY baby it didn't occur to us to check for the first minute or so. We already had names picked out so when we pulled back the little blanket Adam and I simultaneously said "ELLIOT!" Snuggling with my *little baby boy, at home, surrounded by amazing women and my husband, Elliot's dad, was the best moment of my life.*

AFTER THE BIRTH

After a bit more snuggling, I delivered the placenta and had the tiniest of stitches for the tiniest of tears. Elliot came fast and furious (he was born at 5pm on the button. Only 6 hours of labour!) but he was a tiny wee thing at only 6 lbs 7 oz. I went and had a glorious shower while Adam got to snuggle Elliot, then got back into my own bed to snuggle for the night. My mom arrived at 8pm with sushi and prosecco and by then our amazing midwives and doula had left us all cozy in our house, which our doula had completely cleaned. My mom, who had been somewhat skeptical of our home birth plans immediately understood why we'd wanted to try it. All was calm, breastfeeding was (thankfully) going well, and all we had left to do was get to know each other. And, as Adam says, it really was like any other day. At the end, we were cozy at home and the only thing different was the tiny new person who had come to live at our house.

Really. Truly. Bliss.

14. MANAGING PAIN THROUGH CHILDBIRTH EDUCATION OPTIONS

"Consider the possibility that the resistance to the pain and the fear of pain may be more painful than the pain itself. Notice how the resistance closes your heart and fills your body and mind with tension and disease. Keep relaxing the resistance…the tightness..soften around the pain."

– STEPHEN LEVINE

People tend to either run from pain or embrace it. Pain is a difficult human experience to understand as perception varies and level of tolerance is different from person to person and culture to culture. It is also emotionally and physically subjective. Some people handle the emotional aspect of pain better than the physical and vice versa. You don't really know how you will react until you find yourself in a situation where pain is completely unavoidable. Ina May Gaskin said, "I believe that the pain of normal labor does have meaning. The interesting thing about pain is that it is clean. When you are finished experiencing pain, it is over. Labor pain is a special type of pain: It almost always happens without causing any damage to the body." Like everything in life, pain is transient—it does not last. What is so amazing and paradoxical about the concept of pain is that when avoided, you end up dealing with it in a different way or later in time. As a nurse, I found that women who got an early epidural tended to have more pain and recovery after the birth because of the interventions that were used. The patients I worked with who were afraid of the pain of a vaginal delivery and opted for a C-section were always surprised by the amount of discomfort and recovery time this procedure caused in the end.

Pain is difficult to avoid, but suffering is optional. Pain will arise throughout life in different forms such as relationships, addictions, health issues, and child-birth. We have to change our relationship to pain in order to process it properly. Pain can be physical or sensory, emotional or how we feel about a sensation, or cognitive. Cognitive is the judgment we attribute to pain or the expectations, fears, or projections we put on it.

When pain is the enemy, we solidify it. Resistance is where the suffering begins. You have to acknowledge the resistance and any fear that goes along with that. Soften into the sensations, whether they are emotional or physical, and give them space. Bring awareness to any tightness or places you are holding back in life and in birth. When you take away the thoughts "I can't" and you stop fighting the resistance, you are only left with the pain. This is just a physical experience without suffering.

There are many options when it comes to childbirth education classes to prepare you for labor. The pain of labor is the biggest worry, and most women choose to take a course to help them prepare for this. There are a variety of birthing philosophies available, and I am going to discuss a select few that I encountered while working with mothers in labor and delivery. The information given here is directly from the mothers I worked with and from what I gathered myself while pregnant. It will provide enough background so that you can find the best type of class to work for you based on the underlying belief systems. Preparing for delivery takes time, and every mother should feel safe and supported during labor. Women must dive into the transition of motherhood knowing that they did their best preparing their body, mind, and soul for the journey.

Women tend to want to attend one to three classes at the most, but this approach is not enough preparation, especially for the first baby. If you are planning on a natural childbirth, it is absolutely vital to take a long series of classes, and The Bradley Method has the highest percentage of natural births after their course. If this method is not available in your area, ask other course directors if they have produced statistics. Here we will discuss some of the childbirth education classes and pain management options.

CHILDBIRTH WITHOUT FEAR

Childbirth without Fear is the grandfather of all approaches to pain management in labor. This method, which is not as popular today, is based off the following model: when a woman is not prepared for labor or does not know what to expect, she sets herself up for fear-pain-fear cycle, increasing her anxiety. The premise of this course is to reduce the anxiety and fear surrounding birth in order to reduce the pain. Childbirth education movements of the future took this research and aimed to reduce anxiety through preparation in order to optimize normal childbirth.

LAMAZE

Lamaze supports natural labor and birth through controlled breathing and progressive relaxation techniques, which the mother should practice daily. This system believes that labor should begin on its own. The woman is encouraged to walk and move around. There should be continuous support with her throughout the process. All interventions should be avoided if not medically necessary. Women should avoid giving birth on their back and follow the body's urge to push. This method believes that the mother and the baby should not be separated after birth.

THE BRADLEY METHOD

This method of education encourages the father or partner to be involved in the birth and aims for a natural birth with minimal interventions. The method is based on six needs: darkness and solitude; physical comfort, especially in the first stage; relaxation; controlled breathing; and need for closed eyes or rest. The class is significantly longer than others with up to twelve sessions meeting weekly. Focus is on a well-balanced diet, exercise, taking responsibility during pregnancy and birth (remaining informed), education through healthcare providers and books, and relaxation. Nearly ninety percent of mothers who use the Bradley Method do not use pain medication in labor. I personally completed this class with my first birth and have to say that this statistic was entirely accurate. The class was comprehensive. There was a momentum in the learning process between my husband and myself, which helped us both to prepare for the birth. Because there were so many classes, I also felt supported by the group, and we remained friends after our births.

HYPNO-BIRTHING

Hypno-Birthing believes that with the absence of fear or tension, labor and delivery can be relatively pain-free. The method doesn't promise to put you in a trance but more of a dreamlike state. Anxiety is reduced and confidence is increased through continual application of the technique at home before birth. Contractions are called surges, and there is a focus on relaxation through breathing and visualization. Walsh explained that this specific method does not have significant research to back it up, but other methods using hypnosis during labor have shown dramatic reductions in epidurals and narcotics. Many of the patients that I have taken care of have completed this course and had great success during their labor. The class reduced their fears and gave them the necessary skills to remain calm and focused during labor, ultimately having a natural birth in most cases. Other nurses in my field agree with this assessment from a personal and professional point of view.

BIRTHING FROM WITHIN

Birthing From Within courses are custom-tailored to what the parents want to learn and discuss. They encourage the release of fear through birth, art, and journaling. A variety of pain-coping techniques are covered. There is no value judgment placed on medication options for labor. Women are encouraged to find the path that works best for them during birth.

EPIDURAL

If you are birthing at a medical center and know you want to have an epidural, or can't decide, I highly recommend that you discuss it with your nurse early upon arrival. If it is a small hospital, they may not have the staff available to complete the procedure at the time you need it. If it is a larger center and there are one or two anesthesiologists on staff, you still want to coordinate with them to see how busy the floor is or how many surgeries they may be attending. The time between when you are ready for your epidural and when it comes can feel like a century for some women, so talking about it with the staff ahead of time is important. Know that after you get it you may receive Pitocin, if you are already not on it, to enhance the labor.

Most hospitals will not allow you to have this procedure done until you are three centimeters, but I recommend waiting until you are around five to six centimeters or about to enter active labor. If you really want it and wait until you are seven centimeters your pain load will be much higher and it will be hard to sit still long enough for them to finish in a lot of cases. The timing is important because if you receive it too early, it could stall your labor, but if you receive it a little later, it may be just enough pain relief to relax your pelvis for the baby to easily arrive. Some hospitals would not even consider doing it if you are in active labor, or around eight centimeters, depending on how many babies you have had or how fast your labor is going. If you tour the hospital, ask them questions such as how many patients each nurse has (The best centers have a ratio of one nurse to two patients.), if they have an active anesthesiologist on staff, if they provide gas as another pain relief option, and how many of their patients receive epidurals. You also always want to know the C-section rate, especially for the doctor you are using, and compare that ratio to other practitioners or medical centers.

KIRTAN KRIYA AS TAUGHT BY YOGI BHAJAN

This meditation can be done daily during pregnancy, and music to follow along can be found online and on YouTube. The Kirtan Kriya will help to balance your mood and emotions. It will also help to regulate your menstrual cycle, which is vital when you are trying to become pregnant. You can also do it back to back with your partner to combine your energies. It improves the memory and brain function and balances the glandular system. Sit with your legs crossed and spine straight to start. The SA-TA-NA-MA meditation helps to release haunting, limiting patterns of the subconscious mind and prepare a couple for pregnancy. As you chant, imagine energy flowing through the top of your head, or your crown center, and out your third eye, or the place mid-brow between your eyebrows, in an L shape. This helps to circulate your breath and the energy of the sound current.

Eyes: Meditate at the brow point or third eye (Your eyes will look up and in at your forehead.).

Mantra: SA: Infinity, cosmos, beginning. TA: Life, existence. NA: Death, change, transformation. MA: Rebirth.

Mudra: SA: Touch the first (Jupiter) finger; TA: Touch the second (Saturn) finger; NA: Touch the third (Sun) finger; MA: Touch the fourth (Mercury) finger.

Begin the kriya in a normal voice for five minutes; whisper for five minutes; and then vibrate silently for ten minutes. Then come back to a whisper for five minutes and then aloud for five minutes. The duration of the meditation may vary, as long as the proportion of loud, whisper, silent, whisper, loud is maintained. Try it for 11 minutes at first. Music for this meditation can be found online or on You-Tube, which is easy to follow along with. End the meditation by stretching your hands up over your head and shaking them out and then inhaling and exhaling several times.

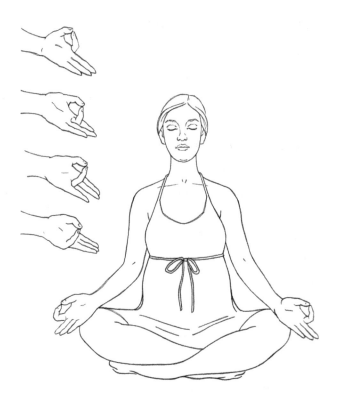

15. CREATING A SAFE AND COMFORTABLE HOME ENVIRONMENT

"Every minute you spend looking through clutter, wondering where you put this or that, being unable to focus because you're not organized costs you: time you could have spent with family or friends, time you could have been productive around the house, time you could have been making money."

–JEAN CHATZKY

Though creating a comfortable home is technically a physiological or base need, it is placed here because while you're pregnant, you will have the desire to nest and create a safe home for your child. I was raised by both of my grandmothers who were very different when it came to the upkeep of their homes and of themselves. My father's mother was always a little disheveled with a chaotic home full of cluttered items. My other Grandma held her home, and her appearance, in the highest regard. Through her I learned the meaning of Obsessive Compulsive Disorder; at the time it wasn't funny, but now it is. I never knew that it was not normal to fold and then refold laundry multiple times or to organize smaller bags in larger ones until I went to college. Through these polar opposite personalities, I was able to come to neutral territory about the organization of a home, the importance of letting go of items not needed, and keeping ones with specific meaning that add energetic movement to areas.

Clutter is anything that is getting in the way of you living the life of your dreams and can take the form of mental thoughts, excess weight, physical items, money, or even relationships. Clutter can be internal or external. Here we are going to focus on the connection between clutter in your home and your overall wellbeing. If your house is constantly a mess, you hold on to items from the past, or you have not completed a spring cleaning—like ever—in your life, it is time to find out the meaning behind your clutter.

I personally had a hard time handling the clutter in my house by myself. My items were a form of safety, and I felt attached and dependent upon them. Even when I took it slowly over a period of weeks, I still felt overwhelmed, especially by the children's toys. I have never been good at asking for help, which is a mechanism of control, but in this case, I hired someone to assist me through the process. It was such a relief to work with a specialist who knew how to approach organizing a house, and it was worth every penny because she helped to create long-lasting results by choosing items to remove and organizing the rest with containers. When I felt attached to an item, I put it in the garage where I couldn't see it, and over time, I found that I completely forgot that I owned it, and it no longer held the same meaning. This is a great way to let things go—separate from them for a while. If you can't afford to hire someone right now, there are many books available that can support you through the process of letting go, getting organized, and feeling grounded in your home.

Kerri Richardson, author of *What Clutter is Trying to Tell You: Uncover the Message in the Mess and Reclaim Your Life*, is one author who has made it her goal to help people clean up themselves and their homes. She suggested that clutter is a form of excess baggage that can sabotage us. Richardson explained that getting rid of the clutter in our lives is a part of a deep healing process where we must let go of patterns from our childhood that we are still literally holding on to. Once you heal the internal emotions, or subconscious issues, you can no longer tolerate the physical clutter around you. When you understand the purpose of the clutter, you can drill down the real source of your problem. Take a look at your home and what it is filled with, and examine what it truly represents in your life. Your items may be weighing you down energetically. For example, if you have issues with your mother or father, but your entire house is filled with photos of them, you are energetically reminding yourself of the pattern and allowing them full stage in the present moment. It may completely uplift the house to take out photos of your dead relatives, because their presence and their items carry a particular frequency.

Clutter is the embodiment of the belief or commitments from the past, which live in a dimensional way in the present. Just as holding too much weight can make you feel heavy and down, too many items in your home can suffocate your radiance and make you small in the world. You may be unconsciously using the clutter to sabotage yourself. So how can you stop and where should you begin? First off, love yourself for where you are at right in this moment. Come to an acceptance that you hold on to things, whether that is items, weight, thoughts, or people. The more you love yourself where you are in this moment, the better you will be able to treat yourself and have the proper motivation to change.

Getting rid of clutter of any sort is difficult because you are navigating new waters and moving out of habits ingrained within you from childhood. According to Richardson, it is all about taking action and making changes approachable enough that we set ourselves up for success. Take it slowly. Break it down to small areas of your house. Rather than asking yourself to clear a whole room or even a closet, start with one cupboard or even part of a counter. When you ease into the project, you can have some success and begin to understand the purpose behind the clutter.

As you begin to de-clutter your life, you may find that your home flows smoother. Take a look at the energy flow of your house. Your environment represents your inner landscape and world. If you are free flowing it may be represented through simplicity, art, or the ability to move throughout the home with ease. The way that you take care of yourself and your home teaches your children a form of self-love and respect. It also creates a great degree of safety and balance within individuals.

EXERCISE:

Go through your house and pay attention to what items feel out of place and energetically off. Remove these items. If you aren't able to give them away, keep them in a separate part of the house for a period of time so that you are able to tell a difference in how you feel when the items are absent. Don't put spring cleaning off until two years from now. Make it a constant habit to give things away. Perhaps you do one section of your house at a time slowly. If you haven't worn or used something in over a year, chances are that you no longer need the item and it is energetically weighing you down.

Richardson Recommends People Do the Following in Order to De-clutter.

1. Begin with identifying what part of your life bothers you the most in regard to clutter. Is it the stack of mail, pile of books, or dirty unorganized cupboards? Maybe even excess weight or thoughts?

2. Complete the following questions via writing: How does it feel when you start to think about those things? Are you irritable, angry, depressed, sad, or overwhelmed? What does the clutter represent about you, your life, and your family's happiness?

3. Once you have a handle on this, go beyond those feelings and listen to what the message from the clutter is saying. Perhaps you need to slow down and take care of yourself or your house. Maybe you feel too unworthy or incapable of taking care of your life even in these small

ways. Possibly you are ready to let go of a relationship or job and your excess clutter is showing up in the physical?

4. Leave the writing and come back later with a deep compassion for yourself. Begin to shift your perspective in the way that you see yourself, and make slow changes that will work for you.

16. TIPS ON HEALING AFTER A CESAREAN AND VAGINAL BIRTH

"I've seen the great force of woman become cheapened, resigned, marginalized, and confused. This to me is one of the greatest crises of all. There is nothing more powerful, more effective or more transcendent than the power of the feminine. Nothing worthy has ever come to bear except for that a woman stood for it to fruit. Woman, you are the beginning and the end."

–GURU JAGAT

As a nurse, I found that many women came in to the hospital expecting a vaginal birth and felt unprepared when they ended up with a cesarean section. For obvious reasons, such as fear, they avoided education on this surgery because they felt it would never happen to them. The average cesarean rate in the United States is thirty-three percent, and sadly this rate is rising there and around the world. The current C-section rate in Brazil is above eighty-five percent in private hospitals. If you have had a C-section, or know another who has, it is important to know how to properly heal emotionally and physically. If you are expecting to have this surgery with your next child, it is also valuable to know how to spiritually prep your body for the event.

Preparing for a healthy and safe surgery, and positively moving on after the experience, is crucial for emotional and physical healing. The key to healing is a complete acceptance of the process. Whether you are preparing for it or it has already occurred, you must let go of the resistance. Most people feel ambivalence or vulnerability when it comes to surgery. If you have had a C-section. or any surgery, in the past, old memories may resurface, especially if you were not completely comfortable with what happened at your birth. The body is able to store these memories in the tissues themselves. Emotions may arise later such as grief, loss, and depression. It is just as important to heal on the energetic level after a surgery as the physical level. Even if you had a surgery years ago you can still heal this area energetically.

The book *Prepare for Surgery, Heal Faster: A Guide to Mind Body Techniques* by Peggy Huddleston is packed full of information for healing after surgery or preparing for one. This guide has been implemented into hospitals all over the United States and is clinically proven to decrease pain and blood loss, and increase the recovery process. Benefits of the program include feeling calmer, use of twenty to fifty percent less pain medication, strengthening the immune system, and saving money on medical bills. The steps are simple, and sometimes obvious, yet no one I know has ever actually taken the time to spiritually prepare, which is disappointing. This book is a good reference for anyone preparing for a C-section.

EXERCISE:

If you know you are having a C-section, have had one in the past, or want to be spiritually and emotionally prepared for the surgery, here are some tips. (This information was taken from Christian Northrup's book *Women's Bodies and Women's Wisdom* **and altered to fit our interests here.)**

I.   **Relax to Feel Peaceful.** Learn how to go into deep relaxation or meditation. This will help improve the immune system and central nervous system, and decrease anxiety. Eighty-five percent of medical problems are associated with stress or unresolved tension or emotional issues in the body. You can buy CDs on this or use my personal favorite type of meditations—Vipassana or Kundalini.

2.   **Visualize Your Healing.** Visualize your ideal surgical outcome, find yourself filled with peace, surrounded by healing light, and in a calm environment.

3.   **Organize a Support Group.** Do you have someone to go into surgery with you and support you through the recovery process? Lose the idea that you are superwoman and can do everything yourself. After surgery you will need to be able to receive from others.

4.   **Meet your Anesthesiologist.** Establish yourself as a patient when you enter the hospital. Get to know them and their values. Even if you are not planning to have an epidural or a surgery, the anesthesiologist should know your medical history and preferences.

5.   **Use Healing Statements.** Here are four healing statements that the medical team should say before surgery. These statements were taken from Christian Northrup's Book *Women's Bodies Women's Wisdom.* And no, it is not odd to ask them to do this—do not get embarrassed. Research has shown that using healing statements reduces complications and healing time, and decreases pain. When your consciousness feels safe, your body will too.

Before the operation you can say the following:

"Following the operation, you will feel comfortable and you will heal very well." *(Repeat five times.)*

After the operation you can say the following:

"Your operation has gone very well." *(Repeat five times.)*

"Following the operation, you will be hungry for _____. You will be thirsty and urinate frequently." *(Repeat five times.)*

"Following this operation, _ _ _ _ _ *(Create a list of positive outcomes.)."*

6. **Use Proper Supplements to Speed the Healing Process.** Always check with your doctor before taking supplements or alternative remedies, especially if you are on medications. You can start taking most of these a week to a month before your surgery to boost your immune system and continue postoperatively. It is best to get as much as you can through natural food sources for absorption.

    - **Vitamin A** to boost the immune system—recommended amount is 25,000 IU a day *(unless pregnant).*

    - **Vitamin C** for collagen synthesis and wound healing—recommended amount is 2,000 mg per day.

    - **Vitamin E** *oil* can be applied to the incision area after the surgical dressing is removed to reduce scarring postoperatively *(Check with your doctor for contraindications.).*

    - **Homeopathy** such as Arnica Montana 30 X *(3 to 4 pellets twice daily)* for swelling and pain.

7. **Create a unique prayer.** Come up with a list of items that are important for your personal healing process. This prayer can be repeated by you and your family members. Some ideas to pray for: a skilled surgery team, your body's positive response, reduced nausea, feeling energized, increased safety, smooth recovery, bowel movements, your spirit to remain high, release of surgery scars imprinted into the body, and returning to regular functioning fast.

TIPS FOR PREPARING AND HEALING FOR A
VAGINAL BIRTH

The healing process for a vaginal birth is not as comprehensive as a C-section, unless there are complications. Before the birth, you can prepare your vaginal canal by stretching it toward the rectum using almond oil or almond oil mixed with a few drops of sandalwood oil. This may not be comfortable for many women as the area becomes hard to reach and may have never been touched like this. If you really want to prepare this area to endure the birth, you can have your partner gently stretch your perineum using two fingers, or you could attempt it while sitting up on the toilet. During pregnancy, walk a minimum of three to five miles daily before birth. This cannot be stressed enough because labor takes endurance and strength. I encourage you to not let your doctor give you an episiotomy during labor and discuss if this technique is ever used beforehand.

After birth the nurse may give you an ice pack which is great for swelling and may provide relief, but the ice-cold sensation can also feel quite shocking to the area if you are not numb from an epidural. An alternative is using warm washcloths to soothe your perineum for the following week or longer (You can alternate between cold for swelling and warm to enhance blood circulation.). Sitz bath herbs can be purchased ahead of time, put in a tea bag, and placed in a crockpot in your bathroom. Add a pile of clean washcloths cut in half. Make sure the crockpot is placed in a very safe and stable place, out of reach of toddlers, and be careful regarding the temperature. Place a thick pad in your underwear, and then place the lightly soaked rag on top to help with pain and healing. You may need to soak the rag with some cold water because of the temperature. This warm rag can also be placed on the perineum while taking bowel movements for support of the area. In the first few days, I recommend taking a stool softener to make bowel movements easier. Kegel exercises should be done before birth and following to maintain muscle strength. Focus on the muscle groups mentally, and tighten them like you are holding in your urine. Do this in short bursts and for longer periods up to ten seconds throughout the day.

A Scheduled Cesarean – Katie's Birth Story

I have always been a bit of medical marvel. Nothing serious or life threatening, more annoying and frustrating. Just enough complications to make sure my parents nailed their 100% insurance coverage every year while I was in high school and college. I'm sure they really appreciated it. Due to my issues, by the time I got married in my early 20's, I was a veteran of eight fairly major surgeries. My parents also should have named me Murphy because if it's gonna happen, it's gonna happen to me. Probably in an incredibly embarrassing way too. Murphy's Law was and still is my constant companion.

Given my medical issues and impressive luck, I shouldn't have been surprised when my gyno discovered I had a little widow's peak at the top of my womb. It has a name and a reason it's there, but I can't for the life of me remember what it's called. Once again, I'm special and my body decided to screw me over. She warned me it could cause a miscarriage, preterm labor or a breech position baby. I wasn't pregnant at the time nor was I getting ready become so, so I didn't give it much thought. Fast forward a year and yay! I'm carrying my husband and I's first little bundle of joy. The little peak thrust it's why back into my life and we watched closely to see what, if anything, would happen. It did. My little girl was hopelessly stuck breech. Even a version at 37 weeks couldn't budge her from her position.

I eagerly awaited my April 22nd scheduled c-section. Surgery obviously doesn't scare me, so I was just excited to have an excuse to miss the pain of natural childbirth and couldn't be called a sissy for it! A little back story on my husband... He's an incredible high school teacher who at the time was the school's Activities

Director. Basically he's was in charge of the school dances, school sponsored events, etc. With a student body around 1300 students, it was a big job. When he learned of my due date (originally April 27), he actually moved the biggest event of the year up a week to avoid it... Murphy's Law, remember? The event is a big fundraiser for Doernbecher Children's Hospital and raises close to $20K a year. Of course, the event was slated for April 21st, the day before my c-section and the big joke around the school office was if I would make it that far and if Mike would be there to direct should I go into labor early. I wasn't concerned, neither was he. No big deal. I didn't want to stay home by myself that evening, so I opted to attend the event. It's a fun evening watching the HS's very best students compete in talents, fashion shows and skits to see who will be crowned Mr. and Ms. Cougar.

I spent the day cleaning, running errands and generally getting ready for our baby girl to arrive early the next day. A good friend of mine, who's husband teaches with mine, joined me at the event that night. She mentioned multiple times that I looked uncomfortable. Of course I looked miserable. I had a human head jammed into my rib cage. She and her husband departed at intermission, so I sat alone in the front row of an auditorium filled with about 500 parents and community members.

With about twenty minutes to go in the program, my cell phone vibrated and I saw my mom calling to let me know they were almost to town and would meet me at my house. I got up to answer it, took two steps and POP!, my water broke. Shit, I only had 12 hours to go before my freaking scheduled c-section! Thank God I had chosen to sit on the classroom side of the auditorium, not the lobby side. I raced up the stairs to the doors, past several students and rushed to the bathroom. It became very obvious I was in a bit of a pickle. My husband wouldn't answer my call likely because he knew I'd be calling at some point to tell him I was headed home. My friend was gone. The school's office manager wasn't answering her cell either. My savior came in the form of one of my husband's students, who I learned later thought I had peed my pants and wanted to make sure I was ok. I quickly told her to go tell my husband my water had broke and

I needed help NOW. Within probably five minutes, students and school staff started pouring into the bathroom, I'm sure convinced they were all about to see a baby born right there at the school. I kept myself locked in the bathroom until both my husband, his secretary and the office manager came to escort me to the car. Mortified at my soaking wet pants, I tried to retain some dignity as I left the bathroom and waddled down the hall to my waiting husband. Fortunately, we were only minutes from the hospital and with all the calls made to my doctors, we arrived. At the wrong door. We had to go through the ER door that late at night. My final shred of dignity gone as I walk, alone, into a packed ER (of course it was packed that night) with soaking wet pants, waiting for my wayward husband to park the car. Contractions I had never expected to feel started up and my temper was starting to heat up as I waited… and waited… and waited for my husband to show up. The nurse waiting to wheel me to the Family Birthing Unit, asked if the gentleman on his phone right outside the door was the one I was waiting for. Good thing I was in pain or I probably would have killed him right there. Seriously? Pretty sure I was more freakin' important at that moment! Get off the damn phone!

Finally, I was checked into a room. I wish I could say I was whisked quickly away to the OR, saved from the pain of contractions. But no. My mother, who had had a blanket made with my daughter's birthdate on it (after all, it was scheduled for the 22nd) convinced them to hold off a little longer, maybe she could still be born on the 22nd, also my oldest brother's birthday. The doctor's arrived, cracking jokes. My husband watched and laughed and made smart alex comments as the contractions came and went. My in laws arrived, more jokes cracked about how impatient both myself and baby girl were. At 11:30PM, I was wheeled away from these crazy people and into the quiet comfort of the room where I would shortly meet my daughter.

My beloved doctor held my hands as the blessed spinal block took away the pains that were getting stronger and stronger. I was so nervous, so excited, so exhausted. My husband came in and sat at my head and we both cracked jokes with the nurses and doctors to try to ease our nerves. They started the surgery not long after and I waited, so eager to hear that first cry. And we waited a little more. I could feel the pressure as they reefed on my stomach. No wonder I had been so miserable... the poor kid's head was literally stuck in my ribs. The pulled and tugged and finally out she came. I will never forget the first words I heard, "Look at those cheeks!" It seemed like forever before I heard that sweet cry as my daughter told us how mad she was at being in the outside world.

More drama ensued during her first week of life. Ladies, breastfeeding is not always best. I may have looked into if my state offered laws allowing mothers to drop their kids off at fire stations and hospitals, no questions asked. And formula is not evil, will not kill your child, make them fat or stupid. My child is lean, wild, beautiful and smarter than her parents most of the time. A true joy in this world. This is the story of how a little girl, hell bent on arriving on her own schedule. Of course my water breaking in front of 500 people, many high school students and then having it announced to them over the PA (Hey, Mr. Huff's wife's water just broke in the front row!) was incredibly embarrassing. Almost as awesome as the night custodian making fun of me still to this day every time I see him at the school. But that's how my life goes. And you just have to roll with it. I can't wait to tell her that story one day. And what's really wonderful, is that we have it all on DVD. You can't ever see me, but you can see the students running back and forth trying to find my husband, then running back to tell the announcers to tell the crowd what had just happened, the crowd cheering and my husband's surprised face as he says he better get going. We watch it every year on her birthday. Oh and if you're wondering, she was born at 12:05AM, April 22nd, making that damned blanket correct about her birthdate.

I had everything planned out. And my daughter laughed from the womb at my plans. The best laid plans are the ones that come crashing down around you. Go with the flow and enjoy it. While some people would have been humiliated, at least I taught a bunch of high schoolers what child birth is really like! You can rest assured that while I await the arrival her sister's c-section, during the same time of year, almost to the day, I will not be attending the event. I think I'll stay home! Thank goodness my husband is no longer the Activities Director!

17. POSTPARTUM DEPRESSION

"When a woman gives birth, the process releases enormous energy for renewal and healing. Something deep within her longs to connect with and heal her own family. If her relationship with them is lacking in some way, this healing feeling will be heightened. The contrast to what could be and what actually is can add to a sense of loss or grief that contributes to depression."

–CHRISTIANE NORTHRUP

After a child is born, feelings, emotions, and physical limits are tested to the extreme. I found that in the hospital the subject of depression was often skipped or just briefly discussed before discharge. Nurses and doctors don't necessarily want to "scare" patients regarding the reality of their new adjustment. The transition into parenthood has been referred to as a developmental crisis, which for some is an opportunity for growth, where everything is new, and it is difficult to know what types of behaviors are normal. Questions regarding postpartum depression (PPD) are vital to discuss for the safety of the mother and newborn. All mothers need to know what it is and how to detect it in themselves and others.

Parenthood brings on a new identity, and the couple must adapt to changes. Some parents may begin to feel a loss if they were unable to complete some of their dreams or had to leave their job. A spontaneous and free lifestyle is no longer a reality because time and energy must be put into this new creation. Even the most confident of women, with no prior history of depression, do not always cope well with these huge lifestyle adjustments. A traumatic delivery or unplanned cesarean section are major causes of distress postpartum leading to depression or fear of labor in the future. Dr. Christian Northrup said, "Postpartum depression is made worse by any sense that the birth was not what the woman hoped for, or that she somehow failed...Labor that doesn't turn out the way you planned can be very traumatic to the mind and body, and women can be left with a type of post-traumatic stress disorder (PTSD)." I have had many patients and friends that were negatively affected by their first birth, so much so that they carried the fear into their next pregnancy and delivery. If your birth does not go as planned or you have a history of a traumatic delivery, please seek help or discuss this with your doctor, friends, and family.

The reality is about eighty percent of new mothers have the baby blues for up to two weeks after delivering. This usually begins between the third and fourteenth day of birth and lasts from hours to weeks. Though it can develop into PPD, with good physical self-care and help around the house, the issues dissipate. PPD can begin anytime from the second week through the first year and last for months. It is distinguished from other types of depression by fluctuations in mood (really good days followed by a bad one). Many women assume that their exhaustion after birth is just the result of sleepless nights; this is often not the case especially if a mother continues to be tired for months. Psychosis (being out of touch, hearing voices, or hallucinating) occurs in one out of every one thousand births. You need to know the symptoms so that you can keep yourself and your baby safe and create a secure foundation for the child's future.

SYMPTOMS OF BABY BLUES

√   **Physical:** Lack of sleep, no energy, changes in appetite, tired even after sleep.

√   **Mental:** Anxiety, worry, confusion, nervousness, sadness.

√   **Behaviors:** Crying, excitability, oversensitivity, irritability.

SYMPTOMS OF PPD (ON TOP OF BABY BLUES SYMPTOMS, YOU MAY SEE SOME OF THE FOLLOWING.)

√   **Physical:** Headaches, numbness, chest pains.

√   **Mental:** Despair, inadequacy, hopelessness, consumed with concern, impaired concentration, loss of interests, thoughts of suicide, bizarre thoughts, feelings of shame.

√   **Behaviors:** Panic attacks, anxiety, new fears or phobias, nightmares, lack of feelings or over-concern for the baby, feeling out of control, extreme guilt.

There are a variety of theories about what causes these postpartum adjustments including thyroid depletion, unrealistic parenting expectations, and hormonal changes. Others believe that childbirth triggers unresolved parental issues. If there are any lingering issues regarding physical, emotional, or sexual abuse that happened in the parent's past, these issues may often arise during childbirth or parenthood in order to be properly healed. Postpartum depression is also magnified when there is a lack of sufficient help around the house. Our society doesn't necessarily condone living in big groups, and many women are secluded after birth. Husbands or partners return to work, and women are left alone to figure out how to raise the baby and keep the household going smoothly, which causes internal stress. Also, when the mother has to separate from her baby too early to return to work, this shock can cause a significant amount of stress for the family.

I trained with Ina May Gaskin, a well-respected midwife in the world, who started The Farm Midwifery center and community in Tennessee. She has assisted in thousands of births and established care with many mothers postpartum. Gaskin surprised me by explaining that she had never seen postpartum depression within her community. She attributed this to the fact that there was no sense of separation and mothers always knew that they had help. Gaskin explained that in parts of Mexico and Central America, women are taken care of for months after birth. Ceremonies include herbal baths, cup massage, and wrapping the mother in fabric up and down her body to "put the edges back on" or reestablish her energy field. This type of care would be wonderful for every mother around the world. Later in the book, an Ayurvedic postpartum method is discussed, which is a great option to reduce the chances of postpartum depression and provide healings.

Assess if you are at risk for postpartum depression: Do you relate to any of the following?

√   Previous history of depression

√   Unwanted pregnancy

√   Unsupportive partner

√   Traumatic birth

√   High expectations for parenthood

√   Being raised by an alcoholic or abusive parent

√   Divorce or separation during pregnancy

√   Major move or life change in the past two years

√   History of moderate to severe PMS

Things to Know for Your Safety:

√   If three or more symptoms are present (over two to three weeks), call a professional (doctor, midwife, prenatal instructor, nurse practitioner).

√   If you see a therapist, make sure he or she is knowledgeable on PPD.

√   Consume adequate amounts of Omega-3 fatty acids.

√   Keep your blood sugar level normal (Low blood sugar exacerbates depression!).

√   Maintain nutritional hormone balance—keep taking a good multivitamin.

√   Think about your expectations after birth. Where did they come from? Your parents, society, yourself?

√   Accept your feelings and try not to judge yourself; you are going through significant changes.

√   Let go of guilt or feelings that it is your fault.

√   Hire help to complete domestic chores.

EXERCISE:

Yogi Bhajan taught that postpartum depression is caused by misaligned pelvic bones that affect a woman's hormones and brain chemistry. Visit a licensed and professional chiropractor before and after pregnancy. Choose someone who has experience working with prenatal and postnatal clients. You can also align your pelvic bones yourself by completing Kundalini Yoga Kriyas, sequences of yogic postures which help to balance the glandular system and bone alignment. You can find these by searching Kundalini Yoga Kriyas for pelvic bone alignment or finding a local instructor.

MEDITATION FOR DIRE DEPRESSION
AS TAUGHT BY YOGI BHAJAN

"This mantra is a declaration of ecstasy, meaning, "We are we, and we are God."
This sound current is so powerful that if you are ever in a dire depression—not
only a depression, but a dire depression – one repetition of this mantra and your
whole mood will start to change. Chant this mantra, and your whole psyche will
change, your energy will change, your flow will change, your mood will change,
your projection and confrontation will change. This is the power of the word."

–YOGI BHAJAN

√   **Posture:** Sit in Easy Pose with legs crossed and spine straight.

√   **Mudra:** Left hand in Gyan mudra with the tip of the index finger
touching the tip of the thumb and the other three fingers straight.
Place this hand six inches in front of the heart center, palm facing the
chest, three fingers held straight and pointing toward the right.

√   **Right Hand:** Make a fist, thumb on top of the bent fingers, index finger
extended straight up. Place this hand about six inches in front of the
right shoulder area. The tip of the index finger should be at the same
level as your eyes.

√   **Mantra:** Humee Hum Brahm Hum. Repeat the mantra loud and clear.
This mantra can be found online. Many wonderful artists sing it and
you can sing with them.

Eyes stay closed with no specific time.

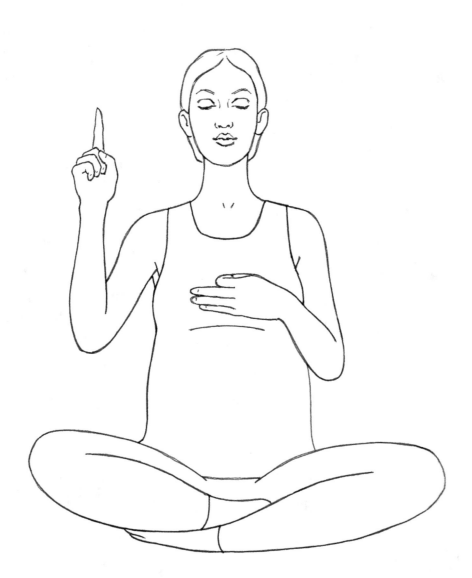

SECTION 3

LOVE AND BELONGING DURING PREGNANCY, BIRTH, AND BEYOND

"If both the physiological and safety needs are fairly well gratified, there will emerge the love and affection and belongingness needs, and the whole cycle already described will repeat itself with this new center. The love needs involve giving and receiving affection. When they are unsatisfied, the person will feel keenly the absence of friends, mate, or children. Such a person will hunger for relations with people in general – for a place in the group or family – and will strive with great intensity to achieve this goal. Attaining such a place will matter more than anything else in the world and he or she may even forget that once, when hunger was foremost, love seemed unreal, unnecessary, and unimportant. Now the pangs of loneliness ostracism, rejection, friendlessness, and rootlessness are preeminent."

–ABRAHAM MASLOW

18. CONNECTING TO YOUR BABY DURING PREGNANCY

"You learn more from hundred twentieth day to the seventh month than you learn in seventy years of your life."

–YOGI BHAJAN

During pregnancy, everything you think, feel, and experience is passed on to your child through the womb. This period is crucial to developing a magical and intelligent individual, and your role is to remain in harmony and balance in order to provide the child with belief systems built on respect, appreciation, and love. If you settled into a daily meditation practice before conceiving, pregnancy is a time to go deeper and expand into greater gratitude and connection. If you have not established a meditation practice and you are pregnant, start now by incorporating any of the techniques discussed in this book. Kundalini Yoga and Meditation is the fastest way to let go of fear, guilt, and insecurities that may otherwise be passed on to your child. During motherhood, you will have to consciously face the belief systems that were passed down through your family regarding nurturing. Your ability to remain stable will be constantly tested by a child capable of bringing all your neurotic tendencies to the surface. As long as you remain awake and aware, any habitual negative parenting behaviors passed down from previous generations can be faced and eliminated. You can heal the past web of expectations, needs, and miscommunication that occurred by taking a deeper look at the way your mother treated you and the way her mother treated her. In order to heal these webs, it is important to not habitually react in the same manner. Time heals all wounds, but the hard and holy work of daily self-psychology and meditation works much faster.

THE IMPORTANCE OF THE 120TH DAY OF PREGNANCY

Though each section of this book is unique and important, I believe that the subject I am going to explain here is by far the most vital and ancient yogic information available to mothers. It is not a mainstream topic, but it will be in future generations. Yogi Bhajan taught that the soul enters the body on the one hundred and twentieth day in the womb, which is around four months. The period up to four months of pregnancy may be an emotional time where the mother feels overweight, insecure, nauseous, excited, and scared. This is the time she must choose to fully accept the soul that will enter her body or not. According to *Creating the Aquarian Child Manual*, the time between conception and the 120th day is when the woman should be consciously meditating and connecting to a high-energy Being still outside her body, making her body and mind as pure as possible, and increasing her radiance through yoga and meditation. This is because she needs to gain as much energy as she can so that on the one hundred and twentieth day, when the soul enters her body, her auric field will be bright and large enough to attract a high vibrational child. There are thousands of souls that want to come to Earth, and they will be battling to make it into a body. On this day a woman must have the highest vibrational frequency to attract a similar energy field. From the 120th day until the day of birth, the mother creates the neuronal patterns that will affect the child for the rest of their life. The time in the womb is by far the most important period of a child's existence because it creates a template that will affect the child's tendencies and patterns for years to come.

It is extremely important to know what day you conceived your child so that you will be able to track which day the 120th day falls on. The day that you have sex or receive in-vitro fertilization and conceive is day one. If you have planned your pregnancy out in the way described earlier in this book, then noting this day should be easy. It gets a little bit tricky when you have been sexually active daily to conceive. Up until the 120th day, you may not want to tell the public that you are pregnant because of attracting unwanted thoughts or energies. An example of this would be a boss that subconsciously does not want you to have a baby and may unintentionally be pulling you back to the office. On the 120th day, you want to feel as beautiful and radiant as you can by meditating, walking in nature, and thinking very positive thoughts. This a good day to have a party surrounded by loved ones and to receive blessings and prayers for your new soul. I have included information on a blessingway ceremony as an option to celebrate and feel like a queen. The 120th day of pregnancy is a time that you can call in a giver, a healer, or a saint. Even if you don't believe this theory, it can't hurt to remain open-minded, feel good, and think positive thoughts around this time or during the fourth month of pregnancy.

AFTER THE 120TH DAY

Up until the 120th day, talk to the soul that you want to bring down, and after that day, speak to the soul that is inside of you. When you communicate with the baby in your womb, make sure to explain what life on earth is like in all details so that the baby feels comfortable when they arrive. You will want to speak to your child throughout the day, and knowing the sex is vital to doing this so you can teach them preferences and relate differently. Give the baby specific details about your schedule, home, neighborhood, chores, relationships, and feelings. Tell them where the grocery store is and who is speaking to you, and explain why you do things in a certain way. Play mantras or soft music for the child. When you do this, you are explaining life on earth to a person who has possibly never been here and who is likely a highly advanced Being.

Yogi Bhajan said, "When a mother is pregnant, the kind of soul she can accept depends on her mental attitude. And then there is another beauty that within the realm of your belly, which is your pregnancy, you can totally transform the soul. The soul is pure and has nothing to do, but the subtle body carries the karma of the previous life. A mother can totally purify the subtle body." The child brings its own personality and karma when he or she enters the womb, but the mother with directed emotion, thoughts and actions can help to clear the path of the child during pregnancy. Meditating during pregnancy will help to do this and so will thinking good thoughts throughout the day. During my second pregnancy, after the fourth month, I began to persistently think about Kundalini Yoga and Meditation, which is something I was not familiar with before. I found the nearest class and went weekly. Without understanding why I was doing it at the time, I compulsively meditated daily and went on to become a teacher of this ancient yogic science following the birth of my baby. The reason I did this is because the soul that entered my body was asking me to. She brought the teachings with her to me and ultimately changed my destiny. Any child who enters a woman will bring their own set of belief systems, energy, finances, and karma that can change the dynamics of the entire family unit. The woman, however, can positively affect the child in the womb and ultimately change the baby's destiny through right actions and thoughts.

THE SEVENTH MONTH OF PREGNANCY

The time between the 120th day and the seventh month is the most important period during pregnancy because it forms the fundamental personality of the child. If the mother is incredibly reactive, the child will likely be too. Any neurosis or glitches in the mother's system will be passed on to the baby especially during this period of time. The people and personalities she is with, emotions she feels, and her environmental surroundings all matter. At the end of the sixth month and beginning of the seventh month is a time when something Yogi Bhajan called the "Acid Bath" occurs for males. During this window, hormones that were once needed in primitive times for hunting and gathering cover the brain. These hormones literally desensitize the male, energetically freeze half of the brain, and create primitive reactions that are no longer required in modern society. The female does not receive these hormones, which makes her more likely to be connected, intuitive, and sensitive. You can help to develop these qualities in the male by completing a specific meditation throughout the pregnancy called the Adi Shakti. The mantra helps the man become creative, less self-centered, and more intuitive in many aspects of life. The meditation can also be done during the pregnancy if you have a girl to enhance the primal power of the Shakti energy and help her to become aware of her destiny. The "Pootaa Maataa Kee Asees" is a mantra you can play during pregnancy and throughout childhood to invoke protection around the child. The mantra "Akal" helps the soul adjust and is important to play in the background after birth to ease the transition. You can choose any meditation or mantra in this book to chant throughout pregnancy. They will all benefit you; however, the Adi Shakti meditation is done for the specific reasons above.

Yogi Bhajan said, "It has been found out that in 60% of all pregnancies the woman suffers physical and mental setbacks. This is quite a serious situation. It has also been found that it doesn't matter how educated our society is, 40% of the children suffer setbacks by an unprepared pregnancy. Normally, there are tremendous changes, which bring deficiency in the character of a child when a woman who is not mentally prepared to handle pregnancy or married life uses the pregnancy and the child as a tantrum to get away from responsibilities. This gives such a weak mind to the child; she damages the child to the extent of making him insecure for up to 60% of the rest of the life." Pregnancy should be taken very seriously as it is a sacred and holy job to bring new souls onto this planet. Don't use your children as an excuse to not live your life fully. If you are reading this book, you are likely ready to do things differently than has ever been done before. A conscious conception and pregnancy is a time of deep internal devotion. To love yourself and another this much is a revolutionary act. If more women began to birth consciously, the entire planet would be affected, because when the woman holds a higher vibration so will the child. Yogi Bhajan said that if women healed their own neurosis and insecurities, within two generations there would be no war on earth. Your frequency matters because the life of the child you are bringing in matters more than you will ever know. Your simple act of self-love and reverence creates a new template that could dramatically switch a familial pattern that has been passed down for centuries. Woman, know thy power.

Call Upon the Maha Shakti

ADI SHAKTI MEDITATION AS TAUGHT BY YOGI BHAJAN

"I feel you must have some time when you are in difficulty. Rather than calling on help from friends and prayer, call the Maha Shakti and see what happens. When India and Indian woman knew this mantra, it dwelt in the land of milk and honey. When they forgot it, it became a hell. Only the forgetting of this mantra has given birth to MTV ... But when a woman knew this mantra she was a living goddess. Without Maha Shakti, God cannot Manifest anything. This is the mantra."

–YOGI BHAJAN, CONSCIOUS PREGNANCY YOGA MANUAL

√   **Posture:** Sit in Easy Pose with your legs crossed and spine straight.

√   **Mudra:** Make fists with both of your hands and extend your pointer finger, or Jupiter finger, out on both hands. The fingers should be pointing straight up and elbows are relaxed against the body.

Time: You can practice this from eleven to thirty-one minutes.

Chant the following mantra: (You can find versions of this music online.)

Adi Shakti, Adi Shakti, Adi Shakti, Namo, Namo

(I bow to the Primal Power)

Sarb Shakti, Sarb Shakti, Sarb Shakti, Namo, Namo

(I bow to the all-encompassing Power and Energy)

Pritham Bhagvati, Pritham Bhagvati, Pritham Bhagvati, Namo, Namo

(I bow to that which God creates)

Kundalini Mata Shakti, Mata Shakti, Namo, Namo

(I bow to the creative power of the Kundalini, the Divine Mother Power)

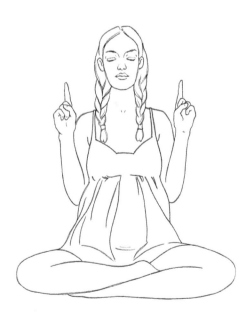

19. PREPARING FOR YOUR BIRTH WITH A BLESSINGWAY CEREMONY

"A Blessingway is an old Navajo ceremony, which celebrates a woman's rite of passage into motherhood. A westernized version of this is the 'Mother Blessing' which is the term I will use out of respect of the Navajo tradition…Unlike a traditional baby shower, where gifts are purchased for the baby, a Mother Blessing is all about nurturing the mother-to-be and celebrating motherhood."

–UNKNOWN

A Blessingway is a wonderful ceremony or pre-birth tradition that is an alternative to a modern baby shower. The ceremony can also be done on the 120th day of pregnancy to bring the soul into the body. It is known as the Mothers Blessing and helps to create a safe and loving environment for the mother with the help of her friends and family members. It is a special way to honor a woman's upcoming birth in preparation for motherhood. Traditionally, it is a woman-only gathering and includes anyone she respects, looks up to, or values for guidance. It helps the woman to prepare herself for birth—emotionally, spiritually, and mentally—and for the all-important role of a new mother. The women circle around the new mother, and she feels safe and held, which is a great way to help her release any fears or blockages in order to come into harmony with the new baby. Often other women will share their birth stories in the hopes of creating an empowering and uplifting environment and better prepare the mother for her own experience. The art of ancient ceremony has been lost, and it is vital that we keep these alternative traditions and ways of connecting alive.

CREATING A RITUAL AT A BLESSINGWAY
FOR THE MOTHER

1: Create a ritual space and form a circle around the new mother.

2: State the purpose of the sacred event in order to shift the space. Set intentions so that the group knows what you are doing and why we are doing it. Everyone should introduce themselves and help the mother-to-be let go of any negative beliefs or fears throughout the ceremony. It is important to hold space and listen while she speaks. Allow the new mother to take her time with the blessings and prayers that are provided by the group.

3: All attention is focused on the mother, and she is pampered and adorned with positive and empowering energies. She is encouraged with personal stories of strength by the group. The Adi Shakti meditation can be completed by the group, or mantras can be played.

4: The ceremony is completed through positive affirmations and good intentions for the world.

5: Share food together in celebration and to ground the energy of the women.

CEREMONY IDEAS

Cord Ceremony: This ceremony is completed by tying the wrists of the women together with a single cord of yarn. The string is kept around everyone's wrists until they hear that birth has started—then everyone cuts the cord as a symbol of unity.

Candle Ceremony: The group can light a candle and pass it around the circle. Each woman offers a word they wish for the mother such as "surrender" or "safety." When the candle reaches the mother, she blows it out, and at her labor, she can relight it to signify a reemergence of these affirmations.

Flowers or Henna: A crown of flowers can be made for the mother by the group, or henna art can be completed on the mother and guests. Henna is not permanent, and there are many kits available on the internet. Adorning women is a lost ancient art that helps to create connection and deep appreciation.

Gift from Nature: Guests are also asked to bring an offering from nature like a small crystal, a feather, or a rock. The item should have significance to them and for the mother. These are offered to the mother and can be placed near her during the birth.

20. AN ALTERNATIVE OUTLOOK ON HOMEBIRTH AND MIDWIFERY

"Birth matters. It matters because it is the way we all begin our lives outside the source, our mother's bodies… For each mother, it is an event that shakes and shapes her to the innermost core. Women's perceptions about their bodies and their babies' capabilities will be deeply influenced by the care they receive around the time of birth… A society that places a low value on its mothers and the process of birth will suffer an array of negative repercussions for doing so."

−INA MAY GASKIN

While working at one of the top medical centers in the country in labor and delivery, in between having children, making a great income, and exploring San Francisco, I had a major spiritual opening that shook my entire world apart. After traveling to India on two occasions, I sat alone in my room before work one afternoon and had a full-blown Kundalini opening which led to five years of deconstructing my life. At the time, I didn't really understand what a Kundalini opening was, but what I knew for sure was that energy so profound and enlightening entered my body, and I was never able to see the world in the same manner again. It was like I went from walking on the streets to standing on a tall building and able to see all the connections of life. The synchronicities that keep us all connected and alive became very clear and palpable.

From that point on, my life was altered, and the next major decision I made was to go study with Ina May Gaskin at The Farm in Tennessee. Gaskin is the most famous midwife in the world and worked tirelessly with a group of women to bring midwifery and natural birth knowledge back into the mainstream (I highly recommend reading her books in preparation for birth.). While studying at The Farm, I learned that birth is a spiritual process that does not need to be filled with fear or interventions, especially for healthy mothers. The midwives at The Farm have delivered well over three thousand babies in the home birth setting with a C-section rate of less than two percent. To put this number in perspective, the average C-section rate in the U.S. is thirty-five percent. The group performed breech deliveries and specialized births, which no other doctor would dare to do, and women from all around the world still travel to The Farm to have their babies because they know they will have a safe delivery without intervention.

Ina May Gaskin told us one of her own birth stories during class one day, a story that ultimately changed her life. During her first birth, all her limbs were tied down, and her baby was "prophylactically" pulled out at high station using forceps (without consent). This was the trend during the time, as C-sections are the trend now. This painful experience empowered her to make changes and become the woman she is today. Meeting Ina May Gaskin created a pivotal point in my life as I began to firmly understand the capabilities of the female during birth and the power of the mind-body connection. Just as her first birth altered the direction of her life, my profound opening created a gateway that empowered me to move forward in my mission to help mothers around the world bring conscious children into this world.

About a month after meeting Ina May Gaskin I became pregnant with my first child and decided that I would have a homebirth using a midwife and doula to help me to deliver. At this time, I also made the choice to leave my job at an acclaimed hospital and return to school to become a nurse practitioner, because I swore I would never tie another woman down to the bed while giving birth again (which is what Pitocin and monitoring felt like to me). All my coworkers were absolutely shocked by my decision to have a homebirth and taunted me with jokes about seeing me in the future for an emergency C-section. My coworkers didn't know that I had begun to see the world much differently because of the events that had happened to me. They also did not know that I was determined to find a conscious and more loving way to bring children onto this planet. Despite my history of witnessing all the tragedies and triumphs that can happen in the birth room, I stuck to my instincts and went ahead with my choice in birthing our child at home.

There were a variety of logical reasons that hospital birth was not my first choice. I have seen firsthand the multiple interruptions that the medical team provides in their rounds, and I believe that these upsetting forces can slow labor. In most medical centers, there is a need to intervene to help a mother progress at the desired rate. A birth plan can't always protect you from the pressures of a medical team insisting that you, and especially your baby, are in need of help. One intervention usually cascades into another. I did not want to be hooked up to monitors, have bright lights shined upon me, walk on cold hospital floors, or be told that I needed synthetic drugs to keep my labor going. I also did not want the opportunity for anesthesia dangled in front of me because I would have taken it, and I wanted to experience birth naturally. Delayed cord clamping was important to me to ensure that my baby received reserved oxygen, and this does not always happen at medical centers. Though I had two girls, I would have been nervous to have a boy at a hospital because of the pressure of circumcision. This is a very common social and medical procedure where the baby's limbs are held down, and with little, if any, pain relief, his foreskin is cut off. There is absolutely no medical reason for this act, which as far as I could tell from witnessing it as a nurse is traumatic, painful, and crippling to the infant. If you are unable to hold your child's limbs down yourself two days after birth and witness the act yourself, do not partake in this stressful event.

There are also many spiritual reasons for choosing a homebirth. I had full faith in the capacities of my body and wanted to feel its power. Birth is sexual and is designed to be, under the right circumstances, a joyous and ecstatic event. It was important for me to be able to walk around freely and to sway and kiss my husband without the fear of someone intruding. I wanted to be connected to the earth and be able to drop my energy down into it like the billions before me. I needed to feel safe and be surrounded by women that I trusted. By choosing a homebirth, I claimed my body as my own.

I delivered my first baby at home successfully and went on to deliver my second baby at home eighteen months later. My first birth was painful, but my second birth was incredibly blissful and euphoric, which I deem to be the result of all the Kundalini Yoga and Meditations I completed during my second pregnancy. I enjoyed relaxing in my own bed and house after delivering my babies because it added a high degree of comfort, safety, and love to the experience. Homebirth is rare. Only one percent of the population has done it, and it is not for everyone. I included information on a homebirth so you will know there are other options when it comes to birthing your child including the fact that midwives are available and a safe alternative. I want to make something very clear though. Whatever type of birth you have is the birth that was meant for you and the way your baby wanted to enter this world. My above experiences, and the choices I have made, are personal to me, and I hold completely different opinions than you do. I am not a cheerleader for natural or home birth. I am just the postman delivering information so that you can research, plan your birth, and remain informed not by propaganda but by intuition. If you want to have a natural childbirth and don't in the end, do not under any circumstances get down on yourself because what happens cannot be changed and should not create another internal problem. All births are sacred no matter what you choose or what happens, which is why I included a variety of different birth stories in this book. You can't go wrong, as you have created life itself. This book is providing you with various perspectives on this holy act including options on the medical professionals you choose.

Midwifery is an ancient art that has been only recently replaced by professional medical obstetrics. In the past, women took care of women during and after childbirth. One common reason for this was because the cervix of the birthing mother closed when she was in the presence of an unknown male figure or in fear. Most midwives tend to approach birth from a more natural perspective and reduce interventions. They also usually support the mother throughout labor. Midwives create a great sense of love and belonging because their training is different than the medical model. If you have a healthy pregnancy, a midwife may be a good option for you to consider and can be found at various hospitals and birthing centers around the country.

EXERCISE:

Here is a list of questions you might want to ask when considering a midwife who works in a hospital, birth center, or at homebirths:

- ✓ Where and how was she trained?

- ✓ What is her experience, and how many years has she been working?

- ✓ How many births has she attended?

- ✓ How does she handle emergencies? (This will vary in different settings.)

- ✓ For homebirth midwives, what is her transfer rate to the hospital, and what precautions or signs arise to make this decision? Does she have backup for emergencies?

- ✓ What do her services include?

- ✓ Does she work with a group of midwives, and are there certain times she is on or off? Who covers for her when she is off or on vacation?

- ✓ How can you contact her, and how does she communicate?

✓ Does she have any experience with complications or stillbirths?

✓ Do you like her, and does she make you feel comfortable?

✓ Would you want her at your birth?

✓ Is she a friend or a professional—or possibly both?

✓ If she is a hospital midwife, does she stay in the room with you during labor, or do the nurses support you?

✓ Why did she become a midwife, and what is her philosophy of care?

✓ Does she encourage participation from the family?

✓ Does she regularly attend conferences and keep up on education? Are her births peer reviewed for decision-making skills?

✓ What are her beliefs on Vitamin K and Hepatitis B shots given after birth? (I highly recommend refusing Hepatitis B if your labs were negative and putting it off until a later date when the child is older if you choose.)

My Personal Birth Story Written in 2014

DECADE

When you came, you were like red wine and honey
And the taste of you burnt my mouth with its sweetness
Now you are like morning bread, smooth and pleasant
I hardly taste you at all for I know your savour, but I am completely nourished

-AMY LOWELL

My Aunt read me this repeatedly as a child, it was one of her favorite love poems. I recently found it in the collection of books she wanted me to have after she died this past year. The poem reminds me of my husband and of our relationship. We have been together for over 10 years – most everything about our relationship has grown slowly over time. As a result we have an incredibly strong and sweet bond. The only thing that wasn't slow is our new baby.

I got pregnant fast! For some reason I assumed it would take a long time – it didn't. We tested to see if I could even get pregnant one month and found out that I could in just one try. Immediately our lives changed, or at least mine did as pregnancy dramatically altered my lifestyle and goals. I track my menstruation by the phases of the moon and I always ovulate when the moon is full. So it didn't surprise me that she decided to come around the March full moon, I knew she would.

I am a labor and delivery nurse who planned a home birth. I attempted to keep an open mind regarding the experience as a result of my profession, but went into labor with the assumption that it could last as long 24 to 36 hours. My labor was about 6- 7 hours. This is fast, like really fast, especially because it was my first birth. My mother, grandmother and aunt had repeatedly told me that when my labor began I was to call the midwife immediately as they also had fast births. As usual, I should have paid more attention to their advice.

I had "pre-labor" for a week before she came. These "warm-ups" were frustrating because it felt like a lot of disappointing false starts. On the day she decided to come I kept convincing myself that I wasn't really in labor. Contractions were coming every 5, 10, or 20 minutes apart. I was looking for more of a pattern – I was looking for something predictable. Of all people I should know that childbirth is never predictable.

That night as contractions began to speed up we turned on some music and lit a few candles. Within an hour or so I could barely move from my position in the house. I just wanted to sit on my husband and grab the couch for support as the intense sensations ripped through me. My moans turned into pure wild animal sounds. We waited to call the doula with the assumption I couldn't possibly be moving this quickly.

But I was, and by the time she arrived my contractions were every 2-3 minutes. The only position I could handle was with my butt in the air because it took the pressure off my perineum. If I moved they came faster, which I knew was not an option as our midwife had not even left the house yet. She assessed me for a couple minutes and immediately called the midwife. When I got up to pee the toilet was filled with bloody show and the mucous plug. As a nurse I knew that this occurred when a patient was about to push. Yet I remember thinking, "I am probably only two centimeters. Oh shit if I am only two centimeters I am going to beg them – actually make them- take me to the hospital to get an epidural." I was most likely about 7 centimeters at this point – just guessing as I had obviously not even been checked yet.

The doula was attempting to fill up the birth tub to help me manage the pain and hopefully slow down the labor so she didn't have to deliver the baby! I crawled down the stairs to the tub and the wild sounds I was producing were getting louder and stronger. My midwife arrived and I began to yell I am pushing!! Cause I was—and with that my water bag burst open.

She asked for just a couple of minutes to set up her equipment. Which was fair, because a home birth requires a lot of preparation – hot towels, bed setup, fresh water, and a resuscitation area. None of this was done, but luckily I had allowed a second doula to be present at the birth for experience and she was able to complete some of these tasks. I wasn't able to have all the candles in the house lit, the music playing, or dip into the hot water. There was just no time for these romantic last minute home birth touches.

I crawled on to the futon in what my husband calls "Pritam's spiritual center" in our house. It is a room full of art we have collected from around the world - Buddha's, mandalas, crystals, and French doors that open to a courtyard with a blooming magnolia tree. My husband sat behind me and held my head in his lap. My midwife checked me and I was 8 centimeters and pushing. So she kept pressure with two fingers on the cervix and minutes later I was complete.

It took me a bit to figure out how to push because I was afraid. Incredible roars were coming from me, sounds that I had no idea I could make! It didn't hurt like the contractions, and I actually felt a lot of relief, but I was afraid that I was going to literally break open. A couple of things crossed my mind: They can't possibly get me to the hospital for that epidural now can they? Maybe I should ask? And… Screw orgasmic births, who the hell has those?

She arrived in about 40 minutes and it was such a beautiful moment. We were both crying as I held her. It was like my heart burst open and broke at the same time. My husband was the most supportive person through the entire pregnancy, supporting me in the decision to have a home birth, and remaining completely calm during the birth. He cut the cord about 45 minutes later and the three of us were tucked into bed by the birth team. We remained there together as a family for about 5 days bonding with our baby. I didn't even leave the house for 2 weeks because all follow up visits were done at home. Having a home birth was incredible. Midwife care is irreplaceable and is truly a form of art. My heart is wide open, present, and patient as I journey into motherhood. She feels like 10,000 puppies in my arms every moment, which is a beautiful feeling.

21. CARING FOR THE MOTHER AFTER BIRTH - FORTY DAYS OF REST AND AYURVEDA

"These days mothers have no time. That's why we want those forty days—not as a punishment. We are asking that for those forty days the mother and child be together so that creativity and values can be established. From the 120th day in the womb to those forty days from birth, the entire character and values of the child are built"

—YOGI BHAJAN

After giving birth, your psychophysiology is as delicate as your baby's, and you are in a special six-week window of healing that requires a significant amount of love and support. The yogic and Ayurvedic systems believe that the first forty to forty-two days after birth equals the next three to forty years of the mother's health, depending on how she spends her time postpartum. The choices a mother makes in regards to support and rejuvenation after her birth are potent and can ultimately affect her health for the rest of her life. The Western medical system and society in general brushes off the significance of this period, which is detrimental to the mother and the baby. It takes time to heal, for the organs to go back into place, and for the energetic system of the female to stabilize. If you take care of yourself well within this period, you will recover in around three to five months. If you do not, you may suffer from exhaustion relapse that can takes years to recover from emotionally, physically, and spiritually.

During the days after birth, the average mother is visited by guests, fed heavy food, and leaves her house on multiple occasions. In the yogic tradition women, are encouraged to stay home for the first forty days to fully bond with their baby. They never let the baby more than nine feet from them because they know it helps to secure the first chakra of the infant and maintain a sense of stability and love for the rest of the child's life. I highly encourage you to do this and rest heavily after giving birth, sleeping for the first three days and resting for the next ten. Next to your bedside table, always keep a large jug of water or herbal teas, nuts, fruit, and small snacks. Keep mantras playing softly. Gently wrap your belly with stretchy material to keep your organs in place. The idea of seclusion after birth is difficult for most women to understand, especially if they have to watch their other children, maintain their house, or return to work quickly. It was hard for me to do this too, but I wish I would have known about the importance of this sacred time after my first birth. When I honored the forty days of bonding and self-care after my second birth, I had a completely different experience that was much more positive and healing.

After my first delivery, like most mothers, I was exhausted and overwhelmed. I also had a difficult time being in bed, and my mind wandered with thoughts that I had so much to do. I found myself on my phone scrolling social media and antsy to get moving. I did not stay at home with my baby, and as soon as I healed began to take her out in public and visit friends. This is because I did not know any better. At the time, I didn't know the importance of properly preparing for the postpartum period. As result of too much activity, I felt exhausted and filled with anxiety. I decided to do it much differently the second time around and came across the ancient knowledge of using Ayurvedic healing foods after birth for a better recovery.

Ayurveda is a system of alternative medicine originating in India that aims to balance the body through dietary, lifestyle, and herbal treatments. In this holistic belief system, after childbirth, the woman is in a state of "Vata" because the empty space left in her abdomen causes an excess amount of the air element in her body and an imbalance to her system. The signs and symptoms of this state include nervousness, anxiety, fear, constipation, dislike of cold, excess thinking or worry, dry skin, and a spacey feeling. Just about every mother I have ever worked with or met can admit to feeling some, if not all, of these symptoms postpartum. To decrease the Vata state, women need a steady routine, warmth, serenity, and nourishment through food and love.

According to *Sacred Window Ayurveda for Mothers and Children*, the best types of foods to feed a woman postpartum are warm, oily, and filled with carbohydrates such as basmati rice. Warm soupy-like textures are best for digestion and replenishing the body. Proteins should come from easily digestible sources such as split mung beans (soaked overnight to reduce gas), and nuts or seeds. Iron-rich fruits such as dates, prunes, apricots, and figs are great after being soaked in water. Fats, such as ghee or clarified butter, should be used in abundance. Vegetables and seasoning such as ginger, cardamom, clove, and fennel are also beneficial. Foods that are dry, cold, rough, or fermented should be avoided immediately postpartum to ensure proper digestion and increase rejuvenation. Women should also avoid coffee, sodas, chocolate, alcohol, raw garlic, and onions because of the effect they have on the baby. Postpartum Ayurveda encourages the use of full fat milk, but you can replace this with almond or goat's milk if you prefer. Heavier foods are brought into the diet slowly after a long period of time. The Ayurvedic system also encourages the use of warm sesame or almond oil massages for the baby and the mother in order to ground the system and decrease gas. The massages also help to relax and nurture the two and make them feel warm and loved.

The mother and infant relationship is symbiotic; when the mother suffers, so does her child. It is just as important to care for the woman as her baby. In American society, new mothers are not acknowledged. After a short stay in the hospital, women are sent home and many do not have their families near to care for them. Most husbands or partners return to work within days, and mothers only receive six weeks of paid postpartum leave. In many cultures across the world, postpartum care is different; the care of the newborn and the mother is shared after birth and made priority. In order to avoid feeling isolation, lack of support, and exhaustion women must set themselves up for success and honor the sacred postpartum period by creating a plan.

When I decided to fully honor the forty days after giving birth with my second child, my entire experience changed. I planned to make this possible, made sure I recruited help to cook Ayurvedic meals, and bought the food supplies needed far before my birth. I also ensured I had someone available to help take care of my toddler so that I would have time to bond with my baby. The self-care and nourishing food grounded me, and I had much less anxiety. Despite eating an abundance of healthy fats, I lost fifteen pounds faster. My breastmilk was abundant and I was able to be present with my baby without my mind wandering. I fully enjoyed the time bonding with my baby by keeping her close and minimizing guests. I avoided taking her out in public at all costs, and if I went outside on a short walk, I kept her covered and close in a sling. I encourage you to make a post-birth plan and consider honoring this sacred time by slowing down and staying home as much as possible to ensure that the nervous system of your new infant remains calm and you heal properly.

EXERCISE:

Here are a couple of recipes taken from *Touching Heaven*, an Ayurvedic postpartum recipe book and planner that can be found in the reference section. These are great recipes for yourself or your friends after birth.

First Days Rice Pudding

This recipe can be served for up to four days postpartum as the primary meal for the mother, should be made fresh daily, and is the best for digestion and nourishment. Bring water to a boil. Rinse rice before adding to boiling water. When rice begins to thicken, add the sugar, spices, and ghee. Cooking time is about four hours, so leave the dish on the stove at a lower heat, and serve warm when thick. Add extra ghee as desired.

16 cups of pure water

1 cup of basmati rice

2 cups of iron-rich sugar such as molasses or dark jiggery

½ cup of ghee

2 teaspoons ginger powder

☐ teaspoon cinnamon powder

½ teaspoon clove powder

½ teaspoon black pepper

½ teaspoon turmeric

½ teaspoon cardamom powder

Sweet Water Lactation Tea

Two parts fennel seeds and one part Fenugreek seeds in large container of warm water

22. WHAT YOU NEED TO KNOW ABOUT BREASTFEEDING

"Imagine that the world had created a new 'dream product' to feed and immunize everyone born on earth. Imagine also that it was available everywhere, required no storage or delivery, and helped mothers plan their families and reduce the risk of cancer. Then imagine that the world refused to use it."

–FRANK OSKI

From my own experience and background in helping many women learn to breastfeed, I have created a "go to" list for new and experienced mothers with the best tips on breastfeeding. This list includes all the information I wish I had been given prior to the birth of my children and has been very valuable to the patients I have worked with and my friends. Despite my background in medicine, when I had my children, I had a lot of unanswered questions, because it takes time and effort. Below you will find information on breastfeeding, bottle-feeding, pumping, growth spurts, and how to handle your baby's fussy periods. Breastfeeding is a sacred time that allows you to bond with your baby. It also provides the very best nutrients for your baby's growth and immune system. If you are on the fence about breastfeeding, attempt it for as long as you possibly can to see how it feels, and then make your decision after researching both the pros and cons.

√   Breastfeeding in the first week: Frequent nursing in the first week is important. During this period your baby may eat up to eight to twelve times in twenty-four hours. Your milk should start to come in around days two to five; before this your baby is receiving nutrition and immunity from colostrum, which is a clear substance. Don't worry, your baby is getting enough to eat as long as you are feeding on demand! Always drink fluid before and after breastfeeding; you may consume three to five liters of water daily.

√   As your milk comes in, you may feel engorged. Use warm compresses and hot showers before feedings and cold cabbage leaf pieces after to support you through the transition. To minimize engorgement, feed often and ensure you have a good latch. Always make sure you have enough pillows around for support, and try breastfeeding in different positions, such as lying on your side. Ensure that the baby does not turn the neck too much, which can hinder the suck and swallow. Make sure your baby's spine is lined up with a straight neck and head, and always latch your baby on to the breast by opening his or her mouth wide; this can be done by gliding your nipple or finger across the child's check gently. Health professionals call this "fish lips," as a good latch is indicated by a suck and swallow sound and a wide-open mouth on the breast. When your baby has a good latch, keep your hand on the back of his or her head gently to keep the baby latched on. Babies tend to pull back, which causes many mothers confusion. Keep your baby in the latched position until the swallowing begins, and ensure there is space for breathing. If you are having problems, make sure to contact a lactation specialist.

√   Breastfeeding in weeks two to six: The baby will continue to nurse eight to twelve times daily. Nurse when the baby shows signs of hunger (stirring, rooting, hands in mouth). Nursing every two hours in the day and every four hours at night is normal. Sometimes the baby may cluster feed in the evenings during a fussy period. After about six to twelve weeks, babies tend to create more of a predictable routine, and nursing sessions are shorter as the baby becomes more efficient. The baby will eventually stretch time between feedings.

√   Feed your baby for a long period on one breast (up to fifteen minutes), and then transfer to the second breast. The long feedings on one side help your body produce more milk and bring in "hind milk" with increased fat content. Burp your baby in between and offer the next breast if possible. If the baby only feeds on that breast for a few minutes, make sure to start on that side with the next feeding. Some mothers use a little pin on their shirt to remember which side they left off on.

√   If you want to store a supply of breast milk for your baby, the best time to pump is in the morning. Pump in the early hours between feedings. It will only take your body a few days to adjust to this change. Check the website Kelly Mom for great tips on breastfeeding and how to store your milk.

√   Your baby will have growth spurts at approximately seven to ten days, two to three weeks, four to six weeks, three months, four months, six months, nine months, and beyond the first year. The growth spurt can last two to three days or often longer; the baby may act fussy during this time and may want to feed up to every hour. If you are breastfeeding, you may feel that you don't have enough supply. Don't worry! Follow your baby's lead and feed on demand in order to increase it.

√   Is your baby acting fussy? Fussiness usually begins around two to three weeks, peaks at six weeks, and is gone by three to four months.

This behavior will usually occur at the same time each day, often in the evenings. Use the five "S" method to soothe your baby: Swaddle, Shush, Swing (small rapid movements), Suck (provide a pacifier or finger to suck on), and place the baby in the Side or Stomach position (The infant can lie across your lap or shoulder, but must be on the back when sleeping.).

√   If you are breastfeeding: It is generally recommended to wait to introduce a pacifier until at least three weeks of age or older. A bottle is best introduced between weeks four through six. If you are having trouble, try different bottles with a slow flow and make sure that someone other than you attempts this. If you plan on breastfeeding exclusively but want to have the option of someone helping with a bottle, keep introducing it to the baby every day or at least every three days. You can pump milk and someone else can provide this. Know that many babies get smart and refuse the bottle from others if they aren't consistently given it.

√   If you are bottle-feeding your baby and using formula, contact your pediatrician as to how much and how often to feed. Over time your baby will take less bottles with more formula in each bottle. In the early months, babies still need to feed on demand.

√   According to Anthony William, science is one hundred years behind and just barely catching up. Breast milk is made up of sugar, so it is vital to eat healthy carbohydrates and fruits while you are feeding your child. Eat foods such as white potatoes, bananas, all fruits, and quinoa. Most doctors encourage a lot of protein, but I encourage you to focus on fruit.

EXERCISE:

You can repeat this throughout pregnancy, while breastfeeding, and during childhood daily to your child: *"Be the greatest person, be a universal person, be vast, live lightly and forgive all, listen, love, learn, excel, live." Yogi Bhajan*

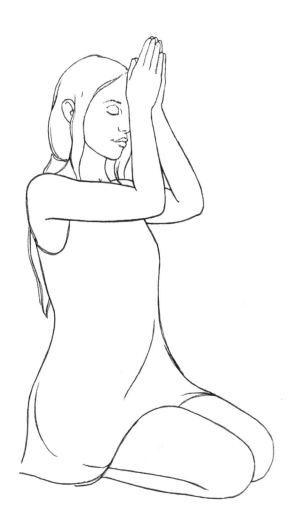

23. PICKING A PEDIATRICIAN
YOU FEEL COMFORTABLE WITH

"The doctor of the future will give no medication, but will interest his patients in the care of the human frame, diet and in the cause and prevention of disease."

–THOMAS EDISON

For some new parents, picking a pediatrician is a daunting task. Your family needs a pediatrician who you can trust, who will listen, and will help support you through the transition into parenthood. It is important to be prepared and ready to ask the right questions in order to find a good match. The search for the right practitioner varies depending on where you live, the amount of time you have, whether you carry insurance, and your belief systems toward medicine.

When I went through the pediatrician search, I was completely shocked by the process, but I also lived in San Francisco where women sign up for preschool while they are still pregnant. True story! I knew there was competition for schools in San Francisco, but I had no idea there was also a lot of stress and very long waiting lists for doctors. It was so competitive that some offices have drawings for new patients, but that is another story. It was important for me to begin searching early and know what type of doctor I preferred.

You should begin your search for the right practitioner early, meaning while you are still pregnant. I would recommend to start three months before your due date. Searches include pediatricians, family doctors, and nurse practitioners. You can always ask your obstetrician or midwife for referrals or go to the American Academy of Pediatrics. This website provides referrals to practitioners who have graduated from an accredited medical school, completed their residency program, and passed the board exam in pediatrics. This doesn't necessarily mean that these individuals have an open heart and open mind though. Make sure that the doctor or nurse practitioner you choose is accustomed to all kinds of parenting styles, is open to listening to your needs, and is neutral with decisions. Make sure you make a list of your family's needs and values so you will attract the right practitioner for your family.

There are a variety of things to look for when finding a pediatrician. Here is a list of questions you might want to consider asking during your search.

√   *What hospitals do you work in?*

√   *For after-hours emergencies, do you meet families outside of the office? If not, who handles this? Where would we go?*

√   *Do you have staff that are available to answer all my questions? How long does it take to hear back from them if so?*

√   *How long is the average wait?*

√   *Who covers for you if you are unavailable or out of town?*

√   *Do you take acute/urgent appointments that day?*

√   *What are your philosophies toward health?*

√   *How do you keep up to date on current medical trends?*

√   *How often are you on call? Weekends?*

√   *What insurance do you take?*

√   *Do you bill insurance?*

√   *Are you ever available for phone consultations?*

√   *How do you feel about vaccinations and alternate schedules?*

√   *How do you treat jaundice or colic in newborns?*

√   *Do you believe in alternative medicine techniques and implement these methods in your practice?*

√   *How do you feel about breastfeeding? Do you ever ask mothers to supplement?*

The Almost Impossible Baby- Sarah's Birth Story

My husband and I had started talking about having a baby, but we weren't sure it was even possible, as I had been diagnosed with a brain tumor five years prior. The doctors said the chemo and radiation to my brain shouldn't have any affect on fertility, but based on my experiences with "should" and "should not," I assumed I would not be able to get pregnant and had decided on adoption for my future children. I am on anti-seizure medication, which increases my risks for birth defects, so that anticipation was another reason for my negative thoughts about becoming pregnant. I found out I was pregnant on an early April evening. I remember having mixed feelings about this- I thought being pregnant was not in my future, we really hadn't been trying, what effects would my medication have on this baby, and was I ready for this adventure?! I also felt like I needed to hide my pregnancy. I didn't feel like I had the struggles and frustrations other women have that make them, in my mind, more worthy of the children they carried. I was worried for my baby. I didn't know what effects my medications would have on the baby and what if, God forbid, the baby died. I decided to share my excitement and blessing selectively.

I was nauseous the first five months. I kept sprite and crackers at work too keep myself going. As a nurse at a school, I was grateful for the cot in my office when I just needed to lie down for a few minutes. I couldn't even fathom how women with more taxing jobs were able to work and be pregnant. I felt like a weenie when I thought about how tired and worn out I felt.

The pregnancy went well until late in the 30th week when I was driving home from work thinking about how often I had felt the baby that day. I realized I really wasn't sure when the last time I felt him move, and called the doctor's office. They had me come in for a non-stress test. The second the monitors were applied to my belly, he kicked. The nurse practitioner decided to do a pelvic exam and a group B strep culture since I was there. During the exam, she discovered I was 1+ dilated and 70% effaced. I was admitted and kept for four days to monitor for further progress of labor. I was able to go back to work with reduced activity.

I was at work at 36 and 6 days when my water broke at about 10:30 am. I wasn't really sure if it had or not, it was a slow trickle and not the giant flood of fluid stereotypical in movies. I called labor and delivery to ask their opinion of the amount of fluid and whether I should come in now or later. Since I wasn't having contractions, they said I could come in now, or wait for a few hours to see how things went. I decided to just go in to be safe, so I called my husband to tell him what was going on. I drove home to get the bag I had packed and my husband.

On our drive to the hospital, my husband took the longest, slowest possible route to get there. I kept laughing at his choices in routes and how stressed he seemed and how calm I was as I still wasn't contracting but was still leaking fluid.

Once we got to the hospital, we checked in at the OB ER. They checked me in and ran tests on the fluid, even though they were sure what it was amniotic fluid.

I was moved to labor and delivery about two or three hours after checking in at 11:30. I told them I wanted to have an epidural when I qualified. I am a weenie when it comes to pain, so I knew I was going to need it. Shortly after, my sister arrived in the room and about an hour later, my parents came. I still wasn't contracting and was dilated to a 4 and 90% so at 4:00 pm they started pitocin. The resident said he thought I wouldn't the baby until 3 or 4 am, but he would come in to check on me about midnight. The contractions were starting and I had to wait for the anesthesiologist to come. I was cranky and not wanting to be in pain, I was given meds to take the edge off. After that, I was aware of the pain but didn't care about it. The anesthesiologist came in and placed the epidural. He did an amazing job and I didn't feel a thing. After that, it was a waiting game

At sometime after the epidural, my in-laws and brother-in-law came too. At this point three of my family and three of his family were there and hanging out. I wasn't feeling contractions but often with the contractions, my baby's heart rate would go down. It wasn't every time, but often enough for me to need oxygen and to be positioned on my side. At about midnight, the resident came in and was surprised I had progressed as much as I had. I was 10 and 100% and ready to push. My doctor was called, and I started to push right when he came into the room. The pediatric team was also called into the room incase my baby needed help after he was born. (If you are counting at this point, there are six family members, three OB team members, three peds team members, a peds nurse, my nurse, and my husband and I in the room. It was a party!) I did push my button right before it was time to push and I was able to concentrate on the pushing and not the pain. The baby's heart rate was still going down and this time it was with every push and contraction. It was a little tense, and my doctor told me I was at a point where I didn't need a c-section to get him out, but they were going to need to use a vacuum to get him out as quick as possible. With the next push, the vacuum was placed and he was born at 12:39 am. The pushing went fast and with the epidural, I could push hard and strong. I tore, and required suturing. Everything I went through, however, was worth it in the end. I have a beautiful, healthy, perfect baby boy and he makes all the nausea, lost sleep, pain, and discomfort worth it in the end.

24. IMPROVING YOUR RELATIONSHIP WITH YOURSELF

"The most terrifying thing is to accept oneself completely."

–CARL JUNG

The most important relationship is the one you have with yourself. When you love yourself, your children will also be vastly affected. All the people in your life are reflections of your past, present, or future and can be utilized as a mirror to understand your state of wellbeing in order to change your vibration to a higher frequency. Ram Dass, a famous spiritual speaker, said, "Your attachment, wishing your loved ones to be different then they are, keeps them the same. Just allow them to be the way they are and love them. Then they may change. But it's not up to you." If you have issues in relationships, it is never really about the other person, it is about your misalignment with your true self and a lack of acceptance of what is. Rather than trying to change the way that other people act, we need to learn to change our thoughts and emotions about the situation and ourselves. We must stop looking outside of ourselves for approval and love, and stop focusing on what other people think of us.

We can gauge our alliance to Spirit or Source by tuning into our emotions, overall mood, and internal sensations. If we are emanating positive feelings such as joy, eagerness, acceptance, and enthusiasm for life, we know that we are going to attract similar experiences. If we are coming from a sense of lack and reside in a state of fear, worry, anger, or frustration, we are going to attract people with similar emotions. Our feelings are our built-in navigation system, which helps us to see if we are out of alignment.

One of the main reasons we become disconnected is because we constantly focus on what we do not want in relationships rather than what we do. Our minds are quick to create separation by acknowledging what other people do wrong rather than what they are doing right. Instead of focusing on all the great traits in individuals, we tend to belittle people by talking about their faults, which are just a reflection of our own insecurities and issues. We are drawn first to the negative aspects of situations because of our natural instincts to protect ourselves. If we do not quickly realign our thoughts to focus on the positive aspects of what we do want to experience in relationships, we will undeniably bring in more of the negative because that is where our vibrational point of attraction is.

Abraham has made it clear that you get what you think about, whether you want it or not, and has changed millions of people's lives from this simple understanding. When you attract relationships that are no longer in alignment with who you really are, these are great opportunities for growth because they offer you a contrast. You cannot know who you really are until you experience who you are not. When a relationship occurs that no longer suits your desires, you can sit with the negativity, or you can choose to expand. Expansion is when you choose to have a new experience that aligns with who you are in the moment and creates a greater potential for joy and creativity.

I had a male friend that I was constantly chasing for attention, and when he did not supply the love I needed, I went into a downward spiral. My focus for a very long time was put on what he was not doing. I was desperate for him to show me love and I waited for him to call or respond to my emails and texts with a heart-breaking neediness like a victim who lost her power. I was more interested in his approval and thoughts about me than how I thought about myself. As a result, I began to attract similar experiences of lack and negativity in other relationships in my life. My friends began to bail out on plans, and I had lack of communication and turmoil in a lot of personal relationships. What I really wanted was to experience love and connection, but I was so deeply engaged in what I was not getting that I created a vortex of negative energy that spiraled into all my personal relationships.

When he did not give the attention I desperately wanted, and all the other relationships in my life lacked true communication, I was fast to place the blame on their behaviors rather than look at my own. What I did not realize is that it was my own thoughts that made me feel bad, not the individual's actions. When I chose to focus my attention on the lack of love, respect, and connection in my life, I got more of that everywhere I turned, which took me farther away from a state of wellbeing. I stuck with this vibration for years, and the more I thought things such as "he doesn't care," "I'm not good enough," "I am alone," and "Everybody wants to fight with me," the more the Universe would provide situations to prove my belief systems. I was attracting the negative vibration I wanted to get away from, which made me feel awful and disconnected.

Abraham said, "When you observe something in another that causes you to feel bad while you are observing it, your negative emotion is an indicator that you are adding to something unwanted". The most important thing we can do is monitor how we are feeling and catch our bad feelings before we get taken into a downward spiral of negativity. When I changed my thoughts about other people, and focused only on positive feelings, I began to change my world. I directed my attention back to myself and realized that it does not matter what anyone else thinks or does. The only thing that matters is how I feel. The only person who was being negative was myself in the relationships because I was choosing to focus on everyone's negative qualities. These experiences showed me contrast and offered me the opportunity to grow by asking for more respect, communication, and love in my personal encounters.

Relationships and experiences should never be thought of us as "good" or as "bad" but as reflection of a part of yourself that can help to launch what you really want in life. You cannot run from one negative relationship hoping that the next one will be better because you will still be carrying the same thought forms throughout. True happiness only happens when you understand that you are responsible for your own feelings. Rather than trying to change my outside relationships, I began to allow people to be who they were. The more I did this, the more I allowed myself to grow into a happier and more loving person. Once I started expanding, by choosing to focus my attention on positive thoughts and emotions, I did not look back to point the finger at what others weren't doing again. I used their ocean of contrast to connect to who I really was and surrendered into the growth

When you are feeling negative emotions toward anything, you are out of alignment. You cannot control the circumstances or the behaviors of other people. You can only control yourself and your personal belief systems and emotions. If you can begin to monitor your thoughts and switch to higher vibrational feelings, you can, without a doubt, change your life and demonstrate how to do this for your children. Every person, place, or thing that you attract into your world is a result of your own asking and vibration. Use these circumstances as a mirror to see yourself more clearly.

EXERCISE:

Wake up in the morning and decide the experience you choose to have for the day. What is the larger experience you want to have in life, with your friends, with your children, and with your family? Personally, I wake up every day and assess where I feel limited because my ultimate goal in life is to keep expanding. In my relationships, I expect to feel trust and respect. With my children, I want to remain in joy and curiosity. Because I set these standards, this is what I receive from the world. What is it that you want to receive? Be specific with your words and emotions.

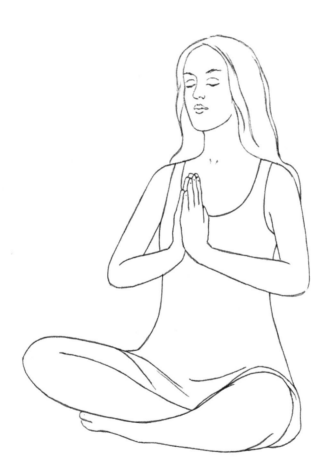

25. VULNERABILITY AND LIVING WITH YOUR WHOLE HEART

"When we spend our lives pushing away and protecting ourselves from feeling vulnerable or from being perceived as too emotional, we feel contempt when others are less capable or willing to suck it up, and soldier on…We let our fear and discomfort become judgment and criticism…Vulnerability is the birthplace of love, belonging, joy, courage, empathy, and creativity. It is the source of hope, empathy, accountability and authenticity. If we want greater clarity in our purpose or deeper and more spiritual lives, vulnerability is the path."

–BRENE BROWN

Webster Dictionary defines the word vulnerability as to wound, capable of being wounded, or open to being attacked and damaged. Vulnerability is taking a huge emotional risk by doing or saying what you feel, which is not for the weak hearted but for the brave. It is stepping out of your comfort zone, following your dreams, and finding your destiny, which, if you ultimately make it there, is serving individuals on a global scale. I believe people who are truly fearless understand what it means to be vulnerable. I don't mean the type of individuals who jump out of planes but those who are willing to totally expose themselves. Many people believe that posting personal information on social networks is a form of vulnerability, but this is not necessarily true. In some cases, this is actually a form of disconnection and a deep-rooted problem in our technologically focused culture. True vulnerability is showing exposure, risk, and uncertainty within yourself to people you trust through open communication. It is doing something that may make you uncomfortable at first so that you can ultimately grow into a better and more loving person. The vulnerable do not run away;, they stay to face the challenge, sadness, or despair to ultimately expand. This is something we need to teach children in order to grow as creative leaders. We are no longer living in a time when people can hide behind their insecurities, weaknesses, or guilt. There is too much to get done, too many individuals who need help, and a planet in desperate need of healing. Vulnerability provides the space to create a sense of love belonging with your friends, family, and children. This is the heart of meaningful human experiences.

Vulnerability is fascinating because it is one of the best roads leading to love, forgiveness, and connection. The fearless are open to vulnerability. One cannot feel true spiritual love when there is any trace of fear inside. Brene Brown, author of *Daring Greatly: How the Courage to Be Vulnerable Transforms the Way We Live, Love, Parent, and Lead,* is an awe-inspiring and leading researcher on the subject. She explained that the vulnerable live *wholeheartedly* and share similar characteristics. They feel worthy of love and belonging and live their lives accordingly. The wholehearted are filled with courage, compassion, and connection. These characteristics shine in all their relationships and are released through positive outlets in their lives. They believe that they are *enough* just the way they are and that vulnerability is a catalyst for positive change.

Brene found that people are drawn to those who can express themselves in this way. Individuals yearn to experience vulnerability through others, but are unwilling to be vulnerable themselves. This is because they are filled with fear when it comes to exposing themselves and repelled by the idea of letting go. She said, "Vulnerability sounds like the truth and feels like courage. Truth and courage aren't always comfortable, but they are never weaknesses…We love seeing raw truth and openness in other people, but we're afraid to let them see it in us. We're afraid our truth isn't enough…" *Why is seeing vulnerability in another being a sign of courage, but a feeling of inadequacy within ourselves?*

EXERCISE:

Below is a list of the characteristics that Brene Brown found in individuals who choose to live their life fully and wholeheartedly. This list contrasts what these individuals are willing to let go of. I recommend printing or copying this list for future reference. Read it out loud replacing the word "cultivate" with the words "I am" or "I am creating." Focus on creating these positive characteristics in your children.

- ✓ Cultivate authenticity: Let go of what people think.

- ✓ Cultivate self-compassion: Let go of perfectionism.

- ✓ Cultivate a resilient spirit: Let go of numbing and powerlessness.

- ✓ Cultivate gratitude and joy: Letting go of scarcity and fear of the dark.

- ✓ Cultivate intuition and trusting faith: Let go of the need for certainty.

- ✓ Cultivate creativity: Let go of comparison.

- ✓ Cultivate play and rest: Let go of exhaustion as a status symbol and productivity as self-worth.

- ✓ Cultivate calm and stillness: Let go of anxiety as a lifestyle.

- ✓ Cultivate meaningful work: Let go of self-doubt and "supposed to."

- ✓ Cultivate laughter, song, and dance: Let go of being cool and "always in control."

26. IT IS TIME TO CHANGE
THE FAMILY PROGRAMMING

"For a person who has not awakened the game is to optimize pleasure and minimize suffering. As you become more aware, you recognize the reality of the Buddha's first Noble Truth: that existence on this plane involves suffering. The more conscious you become, the more you recognize that suffering is how the teaching you need in the moment is coming down."

–RAM DASS

A group of over ten mothers were interviewed by me to discuss issues pertaining to motherhood including concerns with parenting. We ignited their fears and triumphs and created a list for other women to find relief or recognition in. The words isolation, depression, and need for boundaries were repeated many times throughout the conversations, which makes it a vital topic to discuss. The group was yearning for more help and desperate for connection, community, love and belonging. After motherhood the women missed their old selves and the amount of time they had for personal development. Their lives drastically changed after having children; they felt they lost part of their identity and questioned their ability to mother at times. These are common concerns for all mothers but rarely talked about. I remember after having my first baby, I called my friend and said, "Why didn't you tell me how hard this was!" She explained that there is no way to describe it until it happens to you. I disagree. I believe we need to start to talk about the amount of pressure and changes that motherhood brings. The group I interviewed represents the masses and the secrets we keep. Women hide behind perfection to cover weaknesses. Here are some of the general thoughts held by the group that you may feel as a mother at times too. Know, that you are not alone if you ever feel these things.

- ✓ The group felt there was never enough time, especially for themselves.

- ✓ They felt they were alone or that they were the only ones making decisions.

- ✓ They had a hard time making it all work and finding balance.

- ✓ If they went back to work, they were overwhelmed and guilty.

- ✓ If they did not return to work, they felt the exact same.

- ✓ Patience was generally impossible—in stressful moments especially.

- ✓ They were constantly worried about decisions and safety.

- ✓ Some experienced fear of death or leaving their child.

- ✓ They worried they lacked the coping skills to create a healthy family.

- ✓ They held concerns about letting their past rule how they parented.

- ✓ The group wanted more joy and less worry.

- ✓ Their primary frustrations were a lack of time, isolation, lack of resources, and fear of losing independence.

- ✓ They were sometimes depressed, ashamed, and isolated.

- ✓ They wished they had more community and a group of women to turn to.

✓ They mourned their old selves and had a hard time managing emotions.

✓ They all wanted to feel comfortable socially and to be surrounded by similar people in a calm environment where they could find true connections.

This group of women speaks for a nation in need of mothering. Many women have a hard time adjusting into their new role, and it is no surprise as we live in an isolated society. The role of mother is not held in the highest regard and women may feel incompetent at times. There is pressure to perform in so many realms of life, and we multitask to exhaustion. It is time to make life simpler. Stop and tune in. The easiest way to eliminate any confusion around the role of the mother is to fill yourself up to the brim with self-nurturing and take time to explore the pleasures that make you happy. When you are full, you will be much more capable of giving to others. Abundance always boils over with joy. When you become a mother, do no take on a sacrificial role and give up your own passions. Put your oxygen mask on first.

Some of our barriers to acceptance are rooted in past conditioning. When we react to life, we are not actually responding to the moment but to some subconscious patterning buried so deep that we cannot remember why it hurts so much. Yogi Bhajan, the Master of Kundalini Yoga, has said in his lectures that if we were to forgive our mother and father, ninety percent of our problems would be over. Let's make the choice to do this now. Change happens in moments, but pain can last a lifetime. Choose forgiveness and gratitude. It is time to take our eyes inward and see that we are creating our own grief by our negative thoughts. When you begin to think of yourself as not good enough as a mother, catch yourself before the thought goes too far. Always choose a thought that makes you feel good. Focus on what you want to have happen in your life, not on what you don't.

Children teach us to accept life as it is, and they offer us the opportunity to gain mastery over our insecurities, fears, and weaknesses. They remind us that we must always transform, grow, and give up a rigid sense of attachment to the ways things are supposed to be. They do not cause us to feel negative emotions — these feelings were in us all along and are just being magnified. Children come into our lives to help us grow up, as most of us are still children ourselves. It is time to change our communities, and the way we approach parenting through managing our own emotions and creating conscious connections. The general negative emotions and worries surrounding motherhood can be healed through deep inner work, acceptance, and questioning the validity of thoughts.

EXERCISE:

MEDITATION TO RELEASE CHILDHOOD ANGER AS TAUGHT BY YOGI BHAJAN

This meditation will change you completely and will give you subtle powers. If you do it at night, you will wake up feeling amazing.

Posture: Sit in Easy Pose with your arms stretched out straight to the sides. There is no bend in the elbows.

Mudra: Use your thumbs to lock down the Mercury and Sun fingers (pinkie and ring fingers) and extend the Jupiter and Saturn fingers (index and middle fingers). The palms face forward and the fingers point out to the sides.

Meditation: Inhale deeply by sucking air through your closed teeth, and exhale through your nose. To end: Inhale deeply, hold the breath for ten seconds while you stretch your spine up and stretch your arms out to the sides, and exhale. Repeat this sequence two more times.

Time: Complete for three to eleven minutes

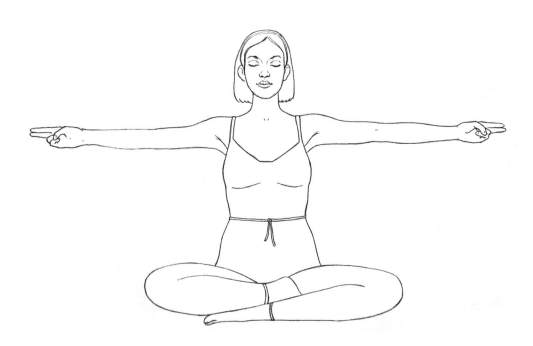

SECTION 4

MEETING ESTEEM NEEDS IN THE EARLY CHILDHOOD YEARS

"A positive self-image and healthy self-esteem is based on approval, acceptance and recognition from others; but also upon actual accomplishments, achievements and success upon the realistic self-confidence which ensues."

–ABRAHAM MASLOW

27. DEVELOPMENT OF THE MAGICAL CHILD

"Matrix is the Latin word for womb. From that word, we get words matter, material, mater, mother, and so on. These refer to the basic stuff, the physical substance, out of which life is derived. The womb offers three things to a newly forming life: source of possibility, a source of energy to explore that possibility, and safe place within which that exploration can take place."

–JOSEPH PEARCE

In the book, *The Magical Child*, Joseph Pearce explained that development is a series of shifts in intelligence that move children from concrete to abstract understanding. This biological plan creates a variety of learning matrices throughout life. Optimally, the child moves on to each stage of development with increased safety, new neural capabilities, and the opportunity to keep building upon past knowledge. Failure in development can happen at any stage, yet life will continue whether proper structural or emotional growth occurred. Pearce completed an exceptional amount of research on what it takes to create a magical child and found that there are certain parental behaviors and choices that can enhance the intelligence of children. This combined with what a child must learn from the

Yogic prospective in development creates a dynamic and alternative way to raise a fulfilled human being. The typical psychological developmental chart starts when the child is born. When researchers begin here, they are missing the most important matrix, the womb.

DEVELOPMENT IN UTERO—A NEED TO REDUCE STRESS

In all the years I dedicated to higher education in psychology, science, nursing, or family practice, I never once came across a course that explained the importance of the time in the womb. The phases of utero growth were discussed, and we had to memorize the critical stages of cognitive development through childhood precisely, but the emotional and psychological affect the mother has on her child during pregnancy was skipped. This is the missing piece to creating a fulfilled and magical child. The womb is the first matrix, and from this space, all is created. Women have not been taught that their thoughts, emotions, and behaviors create the child coming into the world. Missing this vital part of development is one of the biggest problems of our society today.

Pregnancy is a crucial period that affects the capabilities of the child for the rest of his or her life. This time should ideally remain a calm, grounded, and spiritual experience where emotions are kept balanced and environments steady. This can exponentially increase the abilities of the child inside. Though it has not been proven scientifically yet, there is a connection between the amount of stress a mother has during pregnancy and the level of intelligence of the child. Pearce explained, "If the mother's body is producing massive amounts of adrenal steroids during pregnancy, as a result of chronic anxiety, maltreatment, or fear, the infant in the womb automatically shares these stress hormones; they pass right through to the placenta." Hans-Seyle was a nominee for the Nobel Prize for discovering that individuals learn through a balance of stress and relaxation. In stressful situations, adrenaline starts pumping and we go into fight-or-flight mode. When high-stress experiences are over, they provide an opportunity for learning and reflection. We gain muscle memory when the unknown becomes known. If we remain in high-stress, adrenaline-producing, fight-or-flight situations for long periods, our bodies go into chronic stress mode making it difficult to input new information. There must be a period of relaxation for growth or learning to occur. Continued fear, sadness, high work stress, or anxiety can be transferred on to the child in the womb. This is detrimental as it can create an outer world that is the enemy rather than the safe place filled with endless possibility. If you are in a situation that causes you extended stress with little relief while pregnant, you need to make it a priority to remove yourself or relieve your stress, through exercise or meditation.

In addition to reducing stress during pregnancy, it is also important to reduce it at birth. Pearce described a study done with an African tribe who birthed their babies in their village and had very little fear or anxiety throughout pregnancy or at the time of delivery. The infants were born at home, were never separated from their mother, constantly fed by the breast on demand, and always held close in a swing. Researchers found that these infants smiled continuously and with assistance were able to sit up with a straight back and balanced head within days after birth. The average hospital-born infant does not smile, unless it has gas, and is generally listless. These infants were months ahead of European babies in development and sensorimotor skills. They were precocious, advanced, and wide-awake with focused eyes. Blood analyses showed that the infants had none of the adrenal steroids that are typically found as a result of birth stress.

During the time this research was conducted, a European hospital was erected in the region. The babies born in the hospital had none of the extraordinary findings of the ones born under less stress. They were limp, unresponsive, slept heavily, cried while awake, and were much more irritable. This was typical of the hospital-born children I encountered during practice also. The interventions that alter labor progress or significantly drug the mother can cause prolonged stress with no relief during birth. Birthing our children in a village isn't going to work for everyone, but we can take steps to reduce stress during pregnancy and labor.

This book provides ways to do this through meditation, educational birthing classes, doula support, midwives, and fully understanding the environment you are birthing your child in. Reducing stress during childbirth helps to increase bonding between a mother and her baby. Bonding is vital for development and is the next level of the matrix.

BONDING AT BIRTH

Bonding between the mother and baby is a nonverbal form of psychological communication, intuitive response, and telepathic ability to perceive needs. This interconnection is critical in the first hours after birth and is best done with skin-to-skin contact or body molding, prolonged and steady eye gazing, early and continued breastfeeding, smiling, and soothing sounds. Drugs, stress, or exhaustion can negatively affect this period. Separation after birth should not happen under any circumstances unless you or your baby is in critical condition. If you know you are going to have a cesarean section, ensure the hospital allows you to bring the baby to lie near your chest with partner support or be held close to your face. If they don't allow this, ensure your partner is able to do skin-to-skin contact with the baby. Question any hospital policy that says this is not protocol as many medical centers around the world have made this common practice. When you take your baby home, think twice about leaving him or her alone in a nursery, which is essentially a miniature hospital. You are the child's primary matrix and entire world after birth. The infant must be able to learn your face and know under all circumstances that you are dependable, secure, and, most importantly, will always be a point of return from strangers.

Bonding unifies the infant into a new matrix. When it is not completed, intelligence cannot unfold as easily beyond primal needs. This is very important for you to process as a parent. An un-bonded person will spend the rest of their lives searching for someone or something to fulfill the matrix of the mother. When a child is not bonded, they feel abandonment, which creates a neurological pattern that will be repeated throughout their life, reducing their capacity to reach a higher human potential. Pearce explained, "We are never conscious of being bonded, we are conscious only of our acute disease when we are not bonded or when we are bonded to compulsion and material things." It is not uncommon for an un-bonded child to have an –obsessive-compulsive attachment to an item to create a sense of safety. This compulsion, or need for love and security, continues into adulthood and is reflected through unbalanced relationships or a need to look to outside resources for happiness. Everyone knows someone like this or can see parts of this within themselves.

We can look to our culture to see that there are a lot of un-bonded adults running this world. We live in a society that reduces anxiety through the massive consumption of material goods. Individuals commonly live in abusive or manipulative relationships for fear of leaving. Much of social media is based upon reaching out to others for attention and creating relationships that don't really exist. The majority of the world is grasping for something to meet a deep need for love and attachment because this requirement was never met. The bonded child does not require these cultural distractions for inner security and can easily transcend society's norms to contribute something of massive significance for other's happiness. The magical child will have an easier time reaching full potential and will not be held back by limiting beliefs or needs.

UP TO AGE SEVEN

Once your child has reached the age to explore, it is best to allow free play to occur without interruption within a safe environment. Pearce explained, "The greatest learning that ever takes place in the human mind – a learning of such vastness, such reach, such complexity that it overshadows all other learning – takes place in the first three years of life without the child ever being aware of learning at all." Yogi Bhajan also taught that the first three years affects how the child interacts for the rest of their life and builds the fundamental permanent foundation of the character. Their demeanor is generally set after this, so being attentive to their needs and ensuring that they feel understood and loved is vital to development. Most of the learning done in early childhood is through different forms of play including fantasy, imitating, image creation, or transforming objects. Children are still deeply connected to their original Source, and we must do our best not to distort this activity. Allowing your children full freedom to explore and play without engineering learning allows immense growth.

While your children explore, do your best not to interrupt them or impede their growth by projecting constant worry or fear. An example of this would be a mother who worries that her child may get hurt, break something, fall, or get dirty. This mother may interrupt the child while learning a new activity or tasting a new food, projecting her beliefs of whether something is bad or good on to the child. The magical child learns through the silence of neutrality and can form opinions in a safe place with reasonable boundaries. Children take cues from adults on how to behave, and anxiety blocks the expansion of intellect. It is common to have fear as a parent, but it is best not to direct that toward your child's natural behaviors. Children should be able to fully explore nature, get dirty in the mud, or taste food without interruption or interpretation of their experience. The best way for children to grow into unlimited adults with energetic flexibility is through free play and open imagination.

EXERCISE:

Increase Your Child's Development Through the Yogic Perspective:

Teachers from Birth to Eighteen:

√   The mother is the primary caretaker up until the age of three.

√   The father is the caretaker from ages three to seven.

√   At the ages of seven to eleven, extended family and caretakers teach the child.

√   From eleven to eighteen peers teach the individual.

√   Ideally, at the age of eighteen, the child learns from a spiritual teacher. Everyone will meet their spiritual teacher in their lifetime, but eighty percent will run away.

What to Teach Children:

√   **Age Three:** Yogi Bhajan explained that if you don't teach your child prayer by age three you won't have another opportunity. If this is an important behavior to you, start teaching them through example. Sing and tell your children stories based on fantasy and imagination. You can also introduce historical stories. If you don't do this, you risk handicapping your children's happiness. Stories build secure foundations and should be continued throughout childhood.

√   **Age Four:** Teach your child about himself or herself and the world. Tell them stories about the saint, soldier, teacher, or explorer to explain life roles. Role-playing games are important at this age so children know how to act in various situations.

√   **Age Four to Seven:** Teach the child how to create internal balance through ups and downs around the age of five. Martial arts is a good activity to introduce at this age as it enhances spiritual and mental strength and success. Around the age of six and up, the child learns more lessons around trust and kindness. You must teach manners and projection to a child before the age of seven.

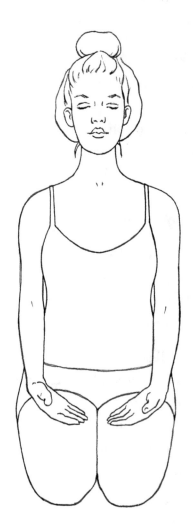

28. BONDING IN EARLY CHILDHOOD

"The truth is, much of what we have traditionally believed about babies is false. We have misunderstood and underestimated their abilities. They are not simple beings but complex and ageless—small creatures with unexpectedly large thoughts."

-DAVID CHAMBERLAIN

The western culture of childrearing has normalized the separation of the infant from the mother to an extent that is detrimental to growth and wellbeing of the child throughout their life. As a culture, if we are going to create an earth filled with individuals who have self-reverence, independence, and respect for others, we must alter the way we bond with our children in the early years. Modern civilization has lost compassion and intuition when it comes to the best ways to raise our babies. Though many hospitals have changed their policy, infants are separated from their mothers at birth for procedures, baths, and mother's sleep time. When parents return home from the hospital, they are encouraged to place their infants in a crib within a separate room and babies are often put on scheduled feedings in order to stretch out meal times. The cry-it-out method is being started at younger and younger ages. This is not the way of our ancestors, and evolution has not prepared the infant for these types of experiences when entering the world. If the child's needs are not met, and expectations go unanswered, babies can easily develop a sense of wrongness or shame about desires right out of the womb. When the infant's needs are met, and they feel security by being held before they can walk, they will grow to have a greater self-esteem and sense of independence as adults.

Jean Liedloff, author of *The Continuum Concept*, went to the jungles of South America on five occasions and lived with a Stone Age Indian tribe, the Yeuana, for a total of two and a half years. During this period, she engaged in their way of living and developed life-changing theories for mothers around the Western world to better raise their children. She noticed that the babies never cried, and as they grew older, the children did not fight or argue among themselves or with adults. Her theories are basic but go against all belief systems we have been taught. First, she argued that during the "in arms" phase, before a child begins to crawl, he or she must be in body contact with the mother or an adult—day and night. Second, when this stage is over, adults must not remain child-centered and should go about their day engaged in their own activities and not be over-devoted to the child. When parents are content and confident in themselves, the child will mirror this behavior in his or her own actions and become self-occupied and happy.

Parents have lost the innate instinctive knowledge of what a baby needs because of the general disconnection that they feel within themselves combined with the patterns they were raised with. After the birth of my first child, I was overwhelmed and had little support or guidance when it came to taking care of an infant and myself. I did not live close to family, and my husband returned to work immediately. It was just the two of us for the first year, and I worked from instincts. My husband and I went against all advice from doctors, friends, and especially family members and let our baby sleep in our bed from the day she was born until she was ready to sleep independently around the age of two to three. At the time I didn't know that this was the "traditional" way to do things in ancient cultures, but I knew for sure that we all slept well, and the arrangement instinctively felt better. I did not have any of the complaints that other mothers suffered from such as exhaustion as my baby slept next to me and was able to breastfeed at night on command with no tears. After the birth of my second child, we continued to co-sleep as a family and for the first few months and made this work with my husband sleeping with our toddler and myself sleeping with the infant in separate beds. This short separation allowed me to heal and bond with the infant in the early months. I also wore my second baby in a wrap on my chest for most of the first six months, which kept her incredibly calm and happy. I didn't know to do this my first time around, and our baby was constantly crying. At the time, I did not understand it, and the crying caused more and more anxiety within me, creating a cycle. I truly wish I would have known what I know now and worn her around my chest from the moment she was born; it would have been a much easier transition.

Co-sleeping wasn't always perfect, and my husband and I had our share of complaining, feet in our face, and discomfort. Despite all this, we had children who slept all night and felt secure and happy. It was also not something that we could comfortably share with all family members or friends because of the reaction we received. Everyone was concerned for the children's safety and kept warning us that is would never end, which hasn't been the case. It felt like separation was the only thing they knew—their mother had separated from them, and hers from her—and it was only natural to start isolation and independence in infancy, because what other option would you have? It is very clear that the world is in desperate need of a change, and at some point, we have to question our society's norms and the traditions that came before us. You must empty yourself of anything that makes you feel limited or puts you in a box in order to find the truth that works for you to create a better family. We cannot continue living out limited belief systems that block our true potential, whether they are related to raising children, self-worth, capabilities, or traditions. Thoughts and beliefs always have an opposite viewpoint. Question those imposing rules you can't live by.

Culturally, co-sleeping is associated with infant death, and this fear far out-weighs the natural benefits of the experience. Dr. James McKenna, a world-renowned infant specialist, explained that the most recent studies showed that bed-sharing infant deaths occurred when an adult had been smoking, drinking alcohol, or taking drugs (illegal or over the counter medicines). Overall, infant death has been associated with at least one independent factor, which might also include a baby sleeping on its stomach, being placed on a pillow, or an extremely obese adult. Experts are beginning to find that co-sleeping can help to develop long-lasting positive qualities in the child such as comfort with physical attention, increased confidence, optimism about life, and an increase in innovation and ability to be alone. Basically, children who co-sleep, or sleep close to their parents in the same room, have the benefits of feeling loved and secure with a greater possibility of growing up to greater emotionally intelligent human beings.

HONORING THE "IN ARMS" PHASE

After living in the jungle for years, Jean Liedloff came to certain conclusions as to why being in constant contact with adults was beneficial to the child during the "in arms phase," which is the time before the child can actively explore the surroundings at about six to eight months of age. Holding the child in these early months kept them passively involved in the group activities of the tribe such as talking, running, laughing, working, or playing. She said, "If he feels safe, wanted and at home in the midst of activity before he can think, his view of later experiences will be very distinct in character from those of a child who feels unwelcome, unstimulated by the experiences he has missed, and accustomed to living in a state of want, though the later experiences of both may be identical." When the baby is held in a wrap close to the chest, he or she is up higher, not lying in a crib or in a carriage, and almost at the level of the faces of those around him. Because of this, the baby can actively assimilate and integrate into the culture they are born into. When they can engage in normal activities of the adults, they experience more sights, sounds, temperatures, emotions, and even the differences between night and day or loud and soft. I believe the key difference between our society is we treat babies and children like they are different from us, and we don't include them in adult activities or treat them as intelligent souls in small bodies. These ancient tribes knew to treat infants with compassion but immediately introduce them to life so they could easily integrate when the time came. These are essential experiences to enhanced growth and development.

In the South American tribe, Liedloff noticed that the adults did not sit and stare at their children, babble, or ask them what they wanted. They were adult-centered and not child-centered. The children were immediately made equals and part of the tribe. They were programmed to become comfortable with life right out of the womb so they could easily maneuver when they were ready. Liedloff also found that holding babies consistently from the time they were born helped them to discharge excess energy from the contact with an active person. When babies are put down in cribs or chairs they often flex their backs and feet while screaming, which could be because they are unable to move around to release the energy they have gathered from food and sun. Babies like action, movement, and bouncing. When you go to the grocery store it is not necessary to give them to someone to watch; instead, take the baby with you in a wrap on your chest and let he or she enjoy your action so that they can also benefit from the movement of energy.

BECOME PARENT-CENTERED

As the children grew older in the tribe, Liedloff noticed that the adults left them alone and kept to maintaining adult-centered activities. They did not fuss, worry, or helicopter over their children because they intuitively knew that they were capable of their own independence and entertainment. Though they occasionally nuzzled their babies, the Yequana tribe was not child-centered. The children were not the center of attention but were always in the midst of adult activities and as a whole were respectful, obedient, cheerful, and happy. In comparison to our culture, this tribe seemed to do things in complete opposite order to ours. We tend to create space from our infants at a young age and then become more child-centered as they grow, which often leads to anxiety over their behaviors. This tribe started out making infants feel secure and part of the community from day one and had very easy children, because as they grew older they treated them like adults.

The modern average mother of a toddler would probably agree that the "terrible twos" is a time of discontent, acting out, and interruption. As children grow, they may become bossy, angry, or rude when they do not get their way and control the adult through intense behavior or crying. In a parent's desire to not be negligent or disrespectful, they often become over-concerned with pleasing their child. When children throw a tantrum, it is easy to bend to their every whim out of desperation, public embarrassment, or a full-on anxiety attack. Liedloff explained that in order to stop this cycle we must center our attention on adult activities that the children can watch and follow along with. This is because the child relies on the parent to remain calm and focused and wants to learn what adults do. When a child visualizes a happy parent, he or she will copy the behaviors and become independent and innovative with personal activity choices. If you are uncertain and unconfident in yourself, and constantly hovering or worrying over your child, it is only natural that your child will try to gain control, and when he or she does so, he or she becomes scared because you are the one who is supposed to be the leader.

When we raise our children to be a part of our tribe from day one and treat them no different than an adult, they grow up respectful, ethical, self-confident, and independent—all attributes of a self-actualized and high-esteemed individual. We have to stop treating children like they are less than us and start demonstrating our own personal power by maintaining control over our own reactions and behaviors. If you offer too much help to children, or constant entertainment through a barrage of activities, you are creating dependence. Through compassion, teach them how to be strong humans by keeping them close after birth but letting them grow when they begin to move forward.

GUIDELINES FOR CO-SLEEPING SAFE WITH INFANTS

Dr. James McKenna stated, "Aside from never letting an infant sleep outside the presence of a committed adult, i.e. separate-surface co-sleeping which is safe for all infants, I do not recommend to any parents any particular type of sleeping arrangement since I do not know the circumstances within which particular parents live. What I do recommend is to consider all of the possible choices and to become as informed as is possible matching what you learn with what you think can work the best for you and your family." I completely agree with this statement and feel that all parents need to go with their instincts, their baby's needs, and the overall family living situation. Here are the basic safety guidelines of sleeping with an infant.

√ Do not smoke, drink, or take any medications (illegal or over the counter) if you want to sleep with your baby. No one else in the bed can partake in any of these activities either. The baby must also have had a healthy gestation with no exposure to cigarette smoke in the womb by the mother.

√ Breastfeeding significantly reduces the chances of SIDS or infant-related death.

√ Whether the infant sleeps next to the mother, in a bed next to the mother, or in a crib, all babies must sleep on their backs, on a flat surface, free from bedding materials, with a light blanket that does not cover their face.

√ Bottle-feeding infants should sleep alongside mother on a separate surface or side bed.

√   Make sure that all adults in the bed are completely aware and comfortable with the infant in the bed.

√   Infants younger than a year should not sleep with younger siblings.

√   Extremely obese individuals or those who can't feel where their body is in relation to another's should not sleep with an infant.

29. SOUND SENSITIZATION OF THE CHILD

"Our greatest adventure is the evolution of consciousness. We are in this life to enlarge the soul, liberate the spirit, and light up the brain."

−TONY ROBBINS

The children who are being born on the planet at this time and into the future are advanced and very sensitive. Just like you are likely different from your parents, consider these children to be light years ahead of you. One of the biggest mistakes parents make is that they consider their children lower than them and treat them as if they are not as intelligent or sensitive to their environment. This is far from the case and is a detriment to the child. Never, under any circumstances, believe that your child does not understand anything, especially when they are unable to speak your language. Yogi Bhajan said,

"When the child is born, you feel that he doesn't know anything, and you know everything. But the fact is, that he knows everything and you know nothing. That is the reality. This is because he has such a powerful instrument of sound reception and for creating sound to communicate his demand. This ability is

lost to the human as he grows in his life. Mothers do not understand this, and they cater to the mood of the child. The child, who is so innocent and unable to know, has what is known as a "sound ring" around him. It is like a musical instrument. The child is there and the bird is flying. He knows and perceives, but he cannot communicate in your language. That does not mean the child is not aware, simply he cannot communicate that awareness."

We have to respect the child's environment and the fact that their sensitivity is very high, especially after birth. It is not what you say but how you say it that matters.

CREATE A SOUND CURRENT OF LOVE

Parents need to start to tune into the sound of their voice and listen to the words that come out of their mouth and the tone that comes with it. Children react differently to the tone of your voice, and they don't necessarily even hear the specific words that you say. It is especially important in the younger years to maintain soft and pleasant sounds in their environment because they are very sensitive. They are very responsive to the sound of your voice because that is the vibration they understood in the womb. Harijiwan, a lifelong student of Yogi Bhajan and teacher of *Creating the Aquarian Child Course*, explained that if you can learn to love your sound current people will love you, and it will give you the power of the Creator. If you monitor your sound, the words that come out of your mouth, and your thoughts, you will literally begin to understand how you influence the world around you. You can do this by listening to the words you speak consciously or even by taping your voice and learning to change your tone with specific people or certain situations. By singing the mantras listed in this book out loud, you can begin to change the effect of your voice and ultimately your life. All of creation comes from sound, and the whole thing is an expression of love. If you create a love experience with your personal sound current, you will manifest your own personal reality and not just be a victim to circumstances.

You can teach your children to do the same thing from a very early age on. From the time they are in the womb to around three years, children are very sensitive to the subtle sound vibrations around them. You need to pay special attention to how you speak to your child, the music that you play, and the people you allow around him or her.

THE SOUND RING

Children are born with what Yogi Bhajan called a "sound ring" around them, which helps them perceive what is happening in a very subtle manner. Just because they don't speak your language doesn't mean that they don't speak their own. At the time of birth, most babies are still connected to deep space, which is why they remain generally sleepy, which can also be considered a meditative state. As time goes on, they begin to perceive the world around them in a manner that you have lost. They likely hear the fluttering of the bird's wing, the sound of breeze sweeping the leaves of trees, and the sound of your cat purring. For all you know, they are speaking with the animals in their very own language. This is because you have lost your sensitivity to the subtle realms and your world has become concrete and dense. To become a conscious mother, you have to begin to perceive things on a new level and become very attuned to the environment that your child is in. Realize how aware your child is of all your interactions and behaviors; you can't hide anything from them because they pick up on everything. The types of sounds that your children hear in the early years will determine how the brain cells activate, so the projection on the sound of the child is very important.

FILL YOUR HOUSE WITH SWEET MUSIC

When your child is born, you can amplify the brain cells and neural connections simply by playing mantras softly in the background of your house at all times. This will help them to thrive. If you don't like mantras or have never heard of them, you can play sweet low-pitched music that the family can enjoy. Avoid putting your child around loud televisions, fighting, obnoxious people, rude talk, or hard rock music. You have the right to remove your child from any situation you consider undeveloped even if it is a family member. Consider all children to be creative and receptive individuals who are always learning what is around them, and from birth to the early years, the way they learn is through the sound current. Because of this, you also want to listen how you speak to your child and monitor how you feel when you talk. There is a big difference between saying, "Get over here, listen to me right now, or else" and "Sweet angel, Mother appreciates it when you listen. Thank you for hearing me."

It is difficult for a lot of parents, including myself, to monitor reactions and not raise our tone with our children when situations become overwhelming. When this happens, parents are reacting from what happened to them in the womb or childhood and likely don't know any better. If you begin to shout at your child, catch yourself and take some deep breaths. Change the sound of your voice and your emotional projection quickly. Yogi Bhajan taught that high punching tones create an electrical storm in the child's brain, which dumbs them down creating great insensitivities and insecurities. Know your breaking point and how much you can handle. My husband and I have set up a signal for when I am at my breaking point and about to lose my temper. When I reach this moment, he takes over which gives me the needed time to cool down and reduce my tone.

With each new birth, the human race is becoming more sensory. The first three years affect how the child interacts with the environment for the rest of their life. Parents must do the very best they can and attempt to not repeat the same patterns they grew up with. You must be very attentive in the first three years in order to build a strong foundation. The child knows everything when they are born and is likely more advanced than you. We must think of ourselves as computers that are decades old and consider our children as the new release. You have to be respectful of how fast their computer runs. This means you cannot patronize your children or speak to them in baby talk. Negotiate with them in an adult manner and listen to their needs. If they are crying, do your best to find out why and speak to them kindly. No matter how adorable they are, treat them as intelligent human beings from the moment that they are born, and see how they will grow into that projection throughout the years.

EXERCISE:

I AM HAPPY MEDITATION FOR CHILDREN AS TAUGHT BY YOGI BHAJAN

"Yogi Bhajan gave this meditation specifically for children to use in times when their parents are fighting and going through a crisis — to give them the experience of remaining stable and unaffected. Of course, the meditation can be done anytime! Children, especially under the age of six, have a much shorter attention span than adults. All meditations with movement and variation work well. They like simple celestial communication."

– HAPPY, HEALTHY, HOLY ORGANIZATION

It can be done by adults too and helps to create confidence in individuals.

Posture: Sit in Easy Pose with legs crossed.

Mudra: In the rhythm of the mantra, the children shake their index fingers up and down (like their parents might sometimes do to make them listen).

Mantra:

I Am Happy, I Am Good, I Am Happy, I Am Good.

Sat Naam, Sat Naam, Sat Naam Jee

Wha-Hay Guroo, Wha-Hay Guroo, Wha-Hay Guroo Jee

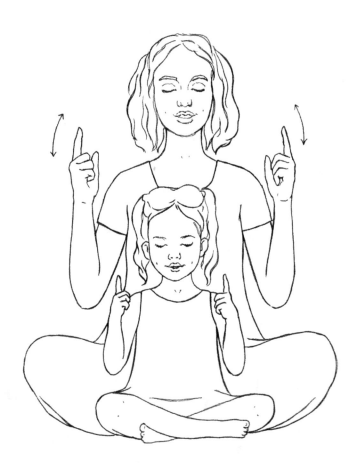

30. CHILDREN GROW BY FINDING PERSONAL PREFERENCES

"Ultimately the person, even the child, must choose for himself. Nobody can choose for him too often, for this itself enfeebles him, cutting his self trust, and confusing his ability to perceive his own internal delight in the experience, his own impulses, judgments, and feelings, and to differentiate them from the interiorized standards of others."

– ABRAHAM MASLOW

Once our basic needs are met, we feel safe and have a healthy sense of love and belonging we can mature into life on greater levels, eventually achieving esteem, independence, and mastery in our endeavors. This type of growth is ongoing, but sometimes individuals can become stuck and continuously cycle through more basic needs instead of going on to higher ones. We all have different views of what growth is and how far we want to go in life. The possibility of growing is always available whether we realize it or not. Many people remain stuck in the comfort zone of repeating the same day over and over again their entire life because it feels safe and they are still dealing with paying the bills, keeping a job, fear of the unknown, or negative relationships. These issues then take precedence over reaching a life of no limits or higher wellbeing. It is easy to get stuck in neurotic tendencies and childhood patterns if we aren't willing to do the spiritual work to release the problems. For a new type of human to live on this earth, one that is full of confidence and ready to rise to the occasion, parents must know where growth can be stunted in the early child-raising years and why. How do the patterns of our childhood and the actions of our elders stop us from being able to experience our highest self? Let's start from the beginning.

Abraham Maslow discussed where growth could be altered in early childhood according to the hierarchy of needs and said that growth only occurs when the next step is more joyous and intrinsically satisfying then the last experience. Development is ultimately the next best thing, and people do it because it feels better and is more fulfilling. It is how we find out as human beings who we are and what we came here to do. Healthy infants live by just Being, which is a state of acceptance and joy. As children get older, they become more spontaneous and curious, and approach their environment with wonder. Maslow states, "Spontaneous, creative experience can and does happen without expectations, plans, foresight, purpose or goal. It is only when the child sates himself, becomes bored, that he is ready to turn to other, perhaps 'higher' delights." We live in a society where we are constantly planning and organizing children's days with activities. We often do not allow them to become bored because we ourselves are frightened of this state. By not allowing boredom, and choosing the best activity we think would suit them, we are not providing the opportunity for them to pick what they want to learn. Thus, impeding their chances of mastering their unique activity and moving on to the next and higher skill. This compulsion to keeping a schedule can easily halt creative expression within the child. Though we believe we are enhancing their growth through activities, we may actually be interrupting it by not allowing the child to unfold at his or her own pace.

Growth takes place in little steps, and it will not occur unless the child feels safe and loved. Then he or she can move up higher on the ladder toward independence and mastery environmental skills. Children operate optimally when they know their security is intact. They want to be able to move forward at any time with the opportunity to retreat if fear arises. If the child has to decide between safety or growth, safety will win hands down in every situation. Think of it as the art of being perfectly imperfect as a parent—allow the child to venture out dangerously in the world and don't intrude. The "don't intrude" part is the most important and often the most overlooked by cautious and protective parents. Stop helicoptering or hovering over your child and avoid planning what they will do next. Once the child feels safe to venture further or go on to another activity, let him or her choose their next move. Children are intelligent people. They are fully intact and capable of making their own choices.

A child begins to gain trust for himself when he is not concerned with the opinions of those around him and is surrounded by a safe, loving, and respecting environment. Not only will a child always choose safety, he or she will also always choose approval when faced with his own growth or making his parents happy. This is because approval and safety are equal. Like many adults, children will sacrifice themselves to feel love. To create human beings who can reach their highest potential, we must have home environments that are accepting, reassuring, praising, admiring, non-comparing, unthreatening, and supporting. This means we have to let go of shaming children when they move forward and use praise instead.

Growth, mastery, and independence arise from safe and loving environments where children are allowed to pick a higher sensation at their own pace. Growth should not be forced but only slightly coaxed or offered in a loving and accepting home. It is easy to impede development when the child does not feel fully accepted by others. Let them be. Let them satiate delights fully and move on to higher and more complex material at their own pace. You don't need to over-plan their lives with multiple classes because it does not allow them to get bored and pick the next best activity to master. When you let go and let them lead, you will increase their sense of self-mastery, self-trust, and, most importantly, self-esteem.

This provides a better possibility for them to continually grow throughout life, stepping off the edge, comfortable with themselves, and into their destiny.

MEDITATION FOR THINKING BEFORE YOU SPEAK AS TAUGHT BY YOGI BHAJAN

"If your lips are not doing a proper job of guarding the most powerful hole in the body (your mouth), do this meditation. Because the lips connect to the Second and Sixth Chakras, you may notice the sex organs and brain being affected"

–YOGI BHAJAN

Next time you are about to interrupt your child or redirect them, try this for three, eleven, or thirty-one minutes.

Posture: Sit in Easy Pose or other meditative posture.

Mudra: Hands are in Gyan Mudra (tip of thumb and index finger touching) resting on knees, elbows straight.

Meditation: In a quick rhythm, like a heartbeat, chant Maa, Maa, Maa, Maa. The lips will tingle.

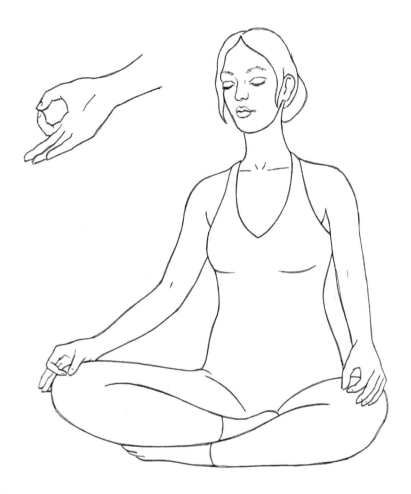

31. PUT YOURSELF IN TIME OUT

"You have no right to tell the child what to do. The child has the right to know what is good and what is bad. If you teach the child good and bad, the child will never leave you. There's no better student. You have never accepted a child as a God-given student. You accept the child as your possession. That's your mistake."

–YOGI BHAJAN

Many parents accept that the time out is the best way to manage their children's unwanted emotions and behaviors. It is what the generations before did so why wouldn't they? Most families across the Western world use this type of enforcement and don't think twice about it, but I am going to suggest that you begin to question the way you discipline your children. Have you ever wondered why we use time outs and where the concept came from? In desperate moments of not knowing better, we need something else to turn to that will teach our children love and compassion.

Through interviews with child specialists, I found that the time out was originally invented by a group of researchers in order to solve the growing problem of juvenile delinquents. The funny thing is, it was never made for the delinquents—it was produced for the parents. When the adult brain is overwhelmed or flooded, the capacity for empathy is reduced. During these moments, it is much easier to put a child in another room than to teach them the emotions that they are feeling. The time out should be a time for parents to take a moment and the family to cool down together. Yet we have let our bull-headed ego get in the way and turned it on to the child, when it is actually us who needs the moment alone. The child is acting developmentally appropriate, and when the adult begins to control, he or she is the one regressing. When we put our child in a room alone, it is only telling them "When you need me the most, you can't come to me. I am emotionally unavailable." This makes it difficult to raise conscious children, who are able to trust the world and the adult taking care of them. When we put children alone to manage uncontrolled emotions, and tell them that they are inherently bad, we are cutting them off from connecting their heads to their hearts.

We need to shift to the family time out, which is really the family putting time in for meditation or a calm break before any reactions occur. We also need to begin to negotiate with our children so they can learn rules of order. Let your child know how the world works before they can speak, and when they start to communicate, teach them how to explain their needs and comprehend that actions have consequences. Children should learn to present their case to you and understand why they should or should not be punished from an early age on. Punishment does not mean neglect or abuse but the fact that every action leads to a sequence of events. Every household will have to decide for themselves the consequences to not following the rules, which may be reduced screen time or toy use. Set up a household system that coincides with the child's level of development when it comes to rules, and use adult language to discuss issues that arise with your child.

When they are two years old, it is most important to contain them during tantrums and teach them to ride the waves of emotions through grounded presence. You can mirror their emotions back to them by saying "Jake is feeling angry...Look how mad Jake is...Grrrrrrr...He wants his toy and isn't getting it." You may need to lower your tone or pitch and create facial expressions to show that you see and feel his or her needs. This teaches children how to connect to their emotions, demonstrates that these feelings pass, and allows them to be seen and heard. If you ignore children's emotions at a young age, you are essentially teaching them to disconnect from themselves and neglecting their opinions. Children must learn that emotions constantly occur but they pass and should not be identified with for long. When they grow a little older, and begin to listen and understand you more, develop a reward system. If your children want something, make sure you negotiate with them on how they can earn it so they learn drive and mastery at a young age. If they do something wrong or go against the rules, let them communicate why they did it and what happened. You want them to be able to communicate both sides of a situation, negotiate their needs, and understand how their behaviors affect others. You also want them to be able to come to you with problems when they get older. If they know that you are levelheaded, trustworthy, and non-reactive, they likely will.

Children have to learn boundaries and consequences, but it is better to do this in a way they can comprehend and develop intelligent emotions. When we become overwhelmed, we have to slow down together. It is time to let our children know there is nothing wrong with them—only something wrong with what they did, reducing the need to create shame. By breathing deeply in front of them and disciplining from a non-reactive state, we can demonstrate presence and teach them patience. If you yell at them, or make a mistake, make sure that you talk about it with them later. Admit when you do something wrong, and explain why you did it so they do the same thing as they grow older.

EXERCISE:

Instead of Putting Your Children in Time Out, Try This Next Time

Meet your child where he or she is at energetically, and project that energy back. Let the child know that you feel their anger or sadness. If your child is having a tantrum, wait a few minutes before trying to communicate. It takes a young child's brain at least ninety seconds to get out of the fight-or-flight response.

They literally cannot understand you or respond in the first couple minutes of a tantrum. So give them a moment, and then let the child know they are heard as their brain adjusts. Get down on their level—physically kneel or sit so the child can see your eyes. After eye contact, give your child a touch and a nod so that he or she knows that you are present. Be clear that you see and feel them and that they are just human beings having a normal experience that will pass. Speak to your children only in a language that has their back so that they know you are always on their side.

Start a New Daily Practice:

Praise your children. Tell your children that you see, hear, and love them. Let them know they are as powerful as the wind, as magnetic as lightning, and as fast as a horse. Make sure they know they can do anything and nothing is impossible, because that is how they will lead a no-limits life. Repeat to them "You are as bright as the sun, brilliant as a rainbow, complete just as you are. You are strong and can do anything in this world because you are God." Boost your children up every morning and every night as a consistent habit, and see how positive their behavior becomes. Children respond to your thoughts about them because thoughts create reality. Make your thoughts and emotions toward your children positive so that you can create a better life.

32. CREATING THE BEST RELATIONSHIP WITH YOUR CHILDREN

"The people in your life will always give you exactly what you expect. No exceptions."

–ABRAHAM

As your child grows older, the simplest way to alter your parenting experience is to focus on what you want rather than what you don't want from your children. This concept can be easily transferred to every relationship in your life. Your opinion and thoughts about your child have a great effect on them and the behavior they elicit. Esther Hicks, channel of the spiritual source named Abraham, was the leader in the new age concept of manifesting by changing thoughts and feelings. Hicks channeled Abraham in the book *The Vortex Where the Law of Attraction Assembles all Cooperative Relationships* and explained, "The more you see things in your child that you do not want to see – the more of that you will see." It is vital to ignore and deemphasize the behaviors that you do not want from your children and praise the ones that you do. The more you discuss, replay, gossip, or think about all the things your children do that you do not like—the more you will enhance and create this unwanted behavior.

Your child is naturally good and connected to Source, but when you try to control him or her through coercion or negativity, you are separating the child from their inner guidance system. Children know how to act, and their behavior is typically normal for their age. It is often the parent's misalignment that is the concern. If discipline is needed, it can be done simply with compassion and lack of shaming. Negotiation will work much better then punishment as they grow up, because it trains them to think not react. When we tell our children they are any different than the way that Source views them, which is always in a positive light, we create discord within them. If we shame or guilt-trip our children regularly, they will naturally begin to change their behavior to please their elders rather than being true to themselves and their own personal likes.

The less we worry and attempt to alter our children's actions, the better. Abraham says, "Contrary to what most parents believe, the less concern they feel for the welfare of their child, the better off their child will be, because in the absence of negative speculation and worry, the child is more likely to gravitate to his own alignment." When we force our children to align with our opinions and actions, we take them away from their own inner knowing. This starts a cycle, which was likely passed down through generations, causing the child to look to others for love and approval. When a family member recognizes that a negative emotion causes disconnection and chooses to pick a more joyous thought and feeling, he or she can stop the generational pattern and ultimately reduce or eliminate illnesses, diseases, and negative experiences.

Parents must work on their own personal vibration first, and then all emotional chaos in their household or relationships will be altered. If parents want to inspire positive behavior in another, they must align with their own personal Source through directed positive emotions and focused thoughts. Harsh discipline does not produce happy or confident children in the long run. In order to change behaviors, we must put all our attention on creating healthy, happy, helpful children. A vision of cooperation will get you farther than a vision of them being negative or naughty.

When we try to change our children's behaviors to make ourselves feel safe, we are creating love based on conditions. Conditional love says, "I love you because you changed yourself so that I could feel happy, and thus you are responsible for the way I feel." Unconditional love comes from just being you—a direct connection to something bigger with no other needs. We can create self-confidence in our children by allowing them the space to make decisions for themselves and showing them how to stay connected by example. Always align yourself first and then interact with your children. Focus only on what you want, make yourself feel good, and see how the world responds. The most important thing that a parent can learn from their child is to stop, look, and listen and be present in every moment. Children understand a lot more than you know; let them lead.

EXERCISE:

MEDITATION TO PREVENT FREAKING OUT AS TAUGHT BY YOGI BHAJAN

"This meditation will alter your energy by changing your nostril breathing. You can't get out of your body, but you can change its energy. If you are thinking something neurotic and find out that you're breathing through your right nostril, start breathing through your left nostril instead. This will change your energy from agni (fire) to sitali (cool). If you are depressed, in a disturbed mental state, start breathing from the right nostril. In 3 minutes you will be a different person. This ability to change nostrils in breathing should be taught to your children within their first 3 years. Exercising this ability can prevent nervous breakdowns. You may work up to 31 minutes."

– KUNDALINI RESEARCH INSTITUTE

Posture: Sit in Easy Pose with your legs crossed with a straight spine and a light Neck Lock (Your neck slightly presses back with chin parallel to floor.).

Mudra: Interlace the fingers with the right thumb on top. Interlace the hands at the center of the diaphragm line, touching the body.

Meditation: Close your eyes. Concentrate on the breath at the tip of your nose.

Notice from which nostril you are breathing. Within three minutes, you should know. If you are breathing primarily through your left nostril, consciously change to your right nostril. Keep your shoulders relaxed and practice changing this breath back and forth for as long as you like.

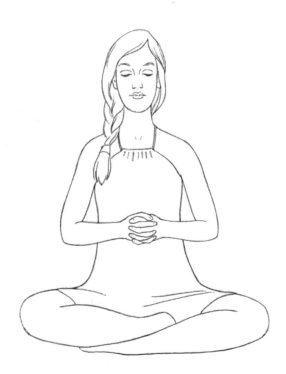

33. MODERN TECHNOLOGY AND THE NEUTRAL MIND

"It has become appallingly obvious that our technology has exceeded our humanity."

–ALBERT EINSTEIN

Technology is growing at a faster rate than ever before, and we are being hit with an increase in thoughts, projections, and information over the internet. Social media and newsfeeds can create a sense of panic in the adult with a low threshold and imbalanced nervous system, often leading to depression and isolation. While studying to become an FNP, there was constant discussion around the use of computers and how much children should be exposed to them. We were trained to encourage parents to reduce screen time during all visits. There is some validity to this claim, and I don't believe we should put our kids in front of a television until midnight; however, we also have to consider that they are more advanced than us and may not have the same sensitization when it comes to technology. Have you noticed how easily babies and small children can utilize an iPhone or iPad, how easily they can change the radio station, and how comfortable they are with technology in general? I recently heard a story of a one-year-old texting her mother's friend back in perfectly readable English. This is because their brain works differently, and they are literally an upgraded version that is likely nothing like us. Just because adults cannot handle how fast technology is running does not mean that the children being born at this time can't either. Letting children use technology will help them to grow, but teaching them how to neutrally navigate the landscape is vital to their survival.

MONITOR WHAT IMAGES YOU POST OF YOUR CHILD

The process of teaching them how to properly manage the sensitization of the internet begins at birth by monitoring what we post on social media platforms. Harjiwan explained during the course Creating the Aquarian Child the consequences of exposing our children on social media at a young age or using their photos to help run business accounts or personal political campaigns. He maintained the stance that children are powerful individuals who should have their rights reserved when it comes to posting their image all over for the world to see. This is especially important when exposing their naked bodies, especially right after birth when they are most vulnerable. Parents are no longer emailing photos of their children out but are using the internet to create updates on their lives. It is natural to want to share your experience and document your children's moments, but as a culture, we have to be more conservative when it comes to protecting our children at times. Social media is a relatively new phenomenon, and we have no idea what the long-term consequences of our choices will have our children's psyches.

I am guilty of this offense and have posted photos of my children's special moments, but I have learned over time that I don't know how far these images are spread or their true effect. I have become more mindful of what I choose to share and with whom. When you know better, you must do better. Essentially that is the point of this book—to teach you how to do your very best by offering an alternative you may have not considered before. If we are going to begin to raise powerful and resourceful individuals who are capable of making their own decisions, we have to protect our children's privacy. We also have to consider how new technology is and how fast it has grown. The television was only invented around one hundred years ago, so we have no idea what the effects of posting photos of our children on the internet will have on their wellbeing or self-esteem later in their lives. As I have said throughout this book, your thoughts matter because they create your reality. If you are posting photos of your child on applications their psyches are naturally going to be affected by the projected thoughts of the masses, negative or positive. Teach them what is appropriate to share with the public and what is not through example. Be cautious and levelheaded with what you project in regards to their bodies and souls. When they are older, they can choose to post what they want and will likely use what you have done as a reference point.

TEACH THEM HOW TO NAVIGATE THE UNIVERSAL WEB

Harijiwan explained during the course that we cannot block our children from the mass amount of information or use of technology, and instead. we need to make sure they develop a neutral mind when it comes to believing opinions and resources. The Berlin Wall only came down a couple of decades ago, and before that, governments were trying to control what people read and consumed. We can't do the same thing to our children. Propaganda is still active, and there are thousands of sources of information publishing varying views of reality. You have to teach them from an early age how to approach this polarity planet with a mind that takes every side into account and is not swayed by outside influence. With a sense of intelligence and self-respect will come a very strong self-esteem and self-concept in who they are and the values they hold. Victory in the modern age is being mentally and emotionally neutral and happy no matter what occurs in the outside world. Neutrality in the face of controversy comes from understanding that for every negative opinion there is a positive one, or there are two sides to every coin.

The vaccination controversy is one of the greatest examples of the importance of doing your own research in order to not to be swayed by varying public opinions. There is always going to be someone who believes that vaccinations are detrimental and another person who would not place their child next to another who has not had the flu shot. You have to read the fine print and come to a decision that feels right to you. This book contains a variety of information and you have to hold enough self-authority to feel what will work in your life and what resonates as truth to you. Teach children self-respect by trusting their intuition and values and not just going with the crowd. Just like you can't force your belief systems on your child, you have to teach them to approach the news and social media with intelligence. This is one of the most important concepts to protect your children in the modern world.

MANAGING THEIR TIME

By encouraging your children to develop their technological skills, I am not encouraging you to allow them to spend the day surfing the web or hide behind a phone. There should always be a natural balance with their time. Utilize your sense of how long they can play with technology while also balancing nature time, activities, and family. You will also have to navigate what type of news is true or dangerous for them to watch. They should know what is going on in the world, but obviously should not be exposed to violence or illicit sex during childhood in any form. If you want to teach your children something, repeat it over and over. If it is important to you for them not to use drugs or drink alcohol, then you could use examples from the social media, newspapers, or movies as a reference point to show them what can happen. If you don't want them posting sexual pictures of themselves, teach them self-love from a young age and how to act by example. You should not project fear in them but come from the heart in an open-minded way to develop the senses, invoke intuition, and create a safe foundation to choose right from wrong. Explain the consequences to them in a language they understand and allow them to ask questions about the world so they know you are the person they can go to when they have problems.

I have done this with my children even before they could speak. I talk to them honestly about the world through my heart, not my head. As a family, we travel with our children extensively, and they have been to many countries and experienced a variety of cultures all over the world. We talk about the details of every city and why things are the way they are openly. I try not to just pass by the homeless man on the street but explain to them why he might be there. Don't lie to your children. If you don't know the answer, find out and explain it to them later. If you build an open and honest communication channel about the realities of the world at a young age, they will know who to go to when they are in need of support far into the future, because when they were little, you didn't ignore their potential or try to keep secrets.

SECTION 5

TEACH YOUR CHILDREN TO LIVE
THE LIFE OF THEIR DREAMS

"Full humanness can be defined not only in terms of the degree to which the definition of the concept "human" is fulfilled, i.e., the species norm. It also has a descriptive, cataloguing, measurable, psychological definition…Among the objectively describable and measurable characteristics of the healthy human species are – 1. Clearer, more efficient perception of reality. 2. More openness to experience. 3. Increased integration, wholeness and unity of the person. 4. Increased spontaneity; expressiveness; full functioning; aliveness. 5. A real self; a firm identity; autonomy, uniqueness. 6. Increased objectivity, detachment, transcendence of self. 7. Recovery of creativeness. 8. Ability to fuse concreteness and abstractness. 9. Democratic character structure. 10 Ability to love, etc."

–ABRAHAM MASLOW

34. THE ROAD TO SELF-ACTUALIZATION AND A LIFE OF NO LIMITS

"Self-actualizing people, those who have come to a high level of maturation, health, and self-fulfillment, have so much to teach us that sometimes they seem almost like a different breed of human beings… It looked like a tendency to do anything creatively…such people can see the fresh, the raw, the concrete … Perhaps more important, however, was their lack of fear of their own insides, of their own impulses, emotions, thoughts."

–ABRAHAM MASLOW

It is reasonable to assume that in almost every human being, or at least in every newborn baby, there is an active will toward good health, growth, and high self-development. We have an impulse toward becoming conscious and fully human individuals, but sadly very few people make it to this type of existence. Somewhere along the way, we are stunted and lose our health, feelings of security, self-esteem, and ability to love, and thus are unable reach our full potential, which is living a life of no limits where we are the creators of our own reality. We all have a no-limit person within us, but we may have lost this as we try to fit into society's, or our family's, view of what and who we are. Those who live without limits are awakened or self-fulfilled and live a happy life regardless of the task they are undertaking. These individuals are self-actualized and fully conscious. They experience the world in total absorption. There are not many of them, and according to Abraham Maslow and other experts, only one in one hundred people make it to this level of living. I am going to make the argument that this number is going to significantly increase in the years to come because there are higher energy children being born on this planet at this time and into the future. If you are reading this book, you are a part of this planetary shift. These children are quite gifted and will have a hard time living by the rules we have established, hence the production of this book for your reading benefit. There are a select few who are on earth right now who are completely and wildly awake, and they have much to teach us. For the rest of the population, the road to self-actualization is a lifelong process, which requires choosing growth daily over fear and repression.

Understanding the human potential by discussing the traits of the self-actualized is one way to comprehend this way of life. The next best thing is to experience it. My goal with this book is to provide your family a road to awakening by presenting optional lifestyle choices and new ways for you to raise your children and your energy. These methods work, and the only thing that is stopping you is your own tendency to fear change and embrace self—sabotage. Know that living as a fully awake human is your natural birthright, and is definitely the natural inclination of children as long as parents don't thwart it. When you begin to experience life in this awakened state, it is like someone turned the lights on in a world of darkness. You will no longer have to chase after anything because you are full. Your abundance, prosperity, and energy will become dynamic and attractive. Synchronicities will create your new reality, and your thoughts will cease to be debilitating. The unknown becomes known, and new worlds open. The density of the body, mind, and spirit fall away to produce light. The self-concept you hold regarding your abilities will be unstoppable because you will become unconcerned with what others are thinking about you. Old patterns disintegrate and you will begin to live out your destiny rather than the life you thought was meant for you. Creativity will begin to flow, and the Universe pours through because you become a muse and a channel. The road to getting here isn't easy, and it isn't always pretty because it takes grace and grit to change. The best gift you can give your children is the opportunity to live this type of existence by allowing them to be who they are without limits so that they can better serve this world.

A self-fulfilled individual carries a set of spectacular and unique characteristics, which Maslow studied during his lifetime so that we could learn from example. His book *Motivation and Personality* described these attributes in great deal and will be discussed here. These individuals listen to their higher selves and do not bring past influences into the present. Their own inner voice is their highest authority and guiding system. They are typically very honest and take responsibility for their life and choices. Each choice he or she makes in life helps to lead to their specific life mission. These no-limit individuals persevere because they have realized their destiny and are much more worried about global issues than personal dramas. Whatever their mission is in life, whether it is a teacher or a dentist, they do it well and become experts in their field.

They trust their own inner tastes and do not look to outside sources for inspiration or acceptance. They also do not feel competition from others because they are driven by their inner world and not a need to meet others' desires. Obstacles on their path only push them forward, and they don't look back. They live by "how they feel" not by "what they think." These people are the highest functioning individuals in our society. They are generally very healthy and keep in shape because it feels good. They reject addictions and tend to stay away from alcohol or drugs. They carry unique attitudes about life and are free from depression. When others may turn to madness, the self-actualized live life with enthusiasm and joy. They don't put limitations on themselves and do not allow others to put any limits on their abilities either. They are commanders of their existence and live without fear, because for them, anything is possible. These individuals hold great esteem for themselves and feel that they belong to the world. They operate on their internal guide and do not need outside individuals' opinions of whether they are taking the correct road. Conscious people like this get out there and do it, and they do it with a sense of humor that is open-minded and original. They are driven and centered in reality, which is based on their own truth.

Maslow explained that these individuals have a vast amount of creative power that serves them to think outside the box. They also tend to have a spontaneous personality that is often childlike because they don't look to the group for approval. Conscious individuals tend to have deep relationships and don't mind spending time alone—they are autonomous in their needs. They live a life full of peak experiences or serene, clear, vivid moments of connection and guidance from a higher source. In these moments, time stands still, and the individual becomes aware of the God-like qualities that he holds within. The difference between the self-actualized and the rest of the world is that these moments of no limitations are common. When they happen, the conscious individual does not walk away feeling fearful or questioning the authenticity of what occurred. They know and believe it as their true self and live unafraid of the great tasks put before them.

You may pinpoint parts of these attributes in your own personality and that is exactly what I want you to do. Rather than focusing on what you are missing, and what you are not experiencing, I want you to begin to focus on all your good qualities and enhance those. Just as parents should focus on the positive qualities of their children, it is important to do the same for themselves. The road to awakening will bring out the best and worst of you to be healed. Stick with all these traits. Enhance the ones that are your strongest attributes, and work with the ones that are not with compassion. In this manner, you can increase your self-concept and self-worth, thus creating a stronger and new pattern in your family system.

SELF-BLESSING FOR SELF-LOVE AS TAUGHT BY YOGI BHAJAN

"Evaluate yourself for three minutes every morning and for five minutes every twilight. You will never miss anything which can serve you or bring you the best. It's eight minutes of self-evaluation. Do it religiously. Evaluate yourself by blessing your head, nose, ears, eyes, mouth, teeth, throat, chest, arms and belly every morning. Just tell them, "Be with me and be nice." In the evening for five minutes, bless your ten toes and fingers, earlobes and top of the ears. It's an acupuncture. Bless every part of the ears and you'll be a new person. You must evaluate and assess yourself. After blessing your body in the evening, bless your good deeds of the day. In the morning bless your good thoughts. Your environments, life, your power, projection and behavior will become the best. You have to bless every part of the body with touch. These are your friends. In the first three minutes, at the dawn of your consciousness, befriend your being physically, mentally, and spiritually. In the evening, befriend your being in detail. This you can teach a three-year-old."

–YOGI BHAJAN

Every night before you go to bed, teach your children to love themselves by blessing their bodies and minds. Say out loud I bless my hands, I bless my heart, I bless my legs, and I bless my mouth, and have them repeat the action. Children learn by example. If you love yourself, they will love themselves. This action brings high self-esteem and self-concept to the children.

35. APPRECIATION IS
THE KEY TO LIFE

"People say that what we're all seeking is a meaning for life. I don't think that's what we're really seeking. I think that what we're seeking is an experience of being alive, so that our life experiences on the purely physical plane will have resonances with our own innermost being and reality, so that we actually feel the rapture of being alive."

–JOSEPH CAMPBELL

Appreciation is the holiest and most sacred feelings that humans can have, and it is vital that you integrate this emotion into your daily life and fully embody it. It holds the frequency of Godliness and equates to love. You must understand and experience this because it is the best indicator of whether you are creating the reality that you want. Appreciation fills your soul with light—it literally feels like your heart is opening in every encounter. When you begin to honor the life forms that surround you, life will begin to honor and bless you back. A state of appreciation is a state of expansion, because from it, all other things will flow. When you are in this state, you will begin to look at the world with innocence and hold a sense of bewilderment of just how wonderful life is. It happens when boundaries drop between individuals and when there is an absence of fear, denial, or hatred. Abraham, the channeled Source of Esther Hicks, explained that appreciation is when you are tuned in and tapped into the vibrational alignment of who you really are, which is God.

Personally, appreciation has been the key to every successful venture or positive change in my life. When I am feeling sad or angry, I always do something, such as exercise, think a better thought, or meditate, in order to change to a higher frequency feeling with the aim of constantly being in a state of appreciation and awe. I do this because when I feel better and am thinking better thoughts, the whole world conspires to assist me in my goals. Feeling appreciation is the end and the beginning for me; it is everything because it makes my world go round. The key to creating the reality that you want is not how you physically feel; it is the thoughts that you think, and the emotions that run through you. If you are feeling a bad emotion, you will tend to start to think negative thoughts, thus creating a vortex of negative experiences. These experiences then become validation for your habitual low vibrational thoughts, which is a nasty cycle to live in. A good example of this would be waking up in the morning, missing your meditation, getting your crying kids out the door, and, in exhaustion, forgetting your bag in the house on the way to their school. This could easily set you off balance, and the next thing you might find is that the woman at the coffee shop is rude and you spill your drink. This turns into an "I told you so" or "see I knew life was out to get me," which isn't the case you are just out to get yourself because you are the creator of your own reality.

Abraham explained that if you aren't feeling appreciation, start with the emotion you are running, and follow it from there to get where you need to be. If you are feeling revenge, you may begin to feel anger; from there, you might feel frustration; after frustration, you may feel hope, and this emotion is in the vicinity of appreciation. When you are in this proximity, pick up your pen and paper and begin to focus on all the things in your life that make you feel happy, whether they are alive or not. Appreciating the little things in your life creates a receptive state of consciousness for more satisfactory things to come to you. When you begin to see the good things, there is a higher tendency for better things to come. Joseph Campbell said it eloquently: "If you do follow your bliss you put yourself on a kind of track that has been there all the while, waiting for you, and the life that you ought to be living is the one you are living. Follow your bliss and don't be afraid, and doors will open where you didn't know they were going to be." You are always surrounded by beauty, but it takes presence and stillness to acknowledge all that is. Babies are naturally in a state of appreciation, and you can see this by the way they interact with their environment through observation and joy.

Appreciation is different than the emotion of gratitude, which is a state of looking at events that happened in your past. When you are appreciative, you are in the present moment looking for what you like best and using all these things as your excuse to attune to who you really are. You could walk down the dirtiest and grungiest street in the city but still see a world full of wonder and awe. Toddlers are always in this state and move from object to object finding a new reality in every moment. This is because they are present, and their minds aren't dwelling in the past or projecting fear into the future. We can maintain this sense of wander with our children by stopping to look at the beauty around us with them and reminding them out loud just how happy we are with the way things are going.

When you are in this state, the world will bend to you because Source will be able to recognize itself within your frequency. You will create tremendously with ease and things will naturally line up. Your friends may not understand why your life is so grand, and they may even begin to feel jealous about how easy everything is for you. When you have reached this point, you have figured out your relationship with yourself and made it your priority. When you are living a life where opportunities arise out of thin air and synchronicities occur to help you meet your goals, you are creating specific thoughts to make these things happen and paying attention to how you are feeling. You must learn to speak and act only from a place of alignment with your higher Source or Spirit. In other words, don't try to fix a fight, write a paper, or have an important conversation without being in alignment beforehand. If you are not in alignment, don't make any major moves. If you are not feeling good and your children are not feeling good, get out of the room and take some space to realign. Put yourself in time out. When people come at you negatively, or you are about to go at them, the best advice I can give you is to just slip away. Come back when you are in alignment and make decisions at that point because you cannot change a problem if you come at it with the same frequency or emotion it started in.

The events that happened in your past, which you call negative, also offer the opportunity for you to feel gratitude. These things happened so that you could become who are today, and any events that you feel were traumatic or destructive hold the same amount of light as your best memories because it is all holy—the whole story is sacred. If your mother was a tyrant, be grateful. She offered you a place to grow from. Whether you had a traumatic childhood or have convinced yourself that you did when you really didn't, it does not matter. It all holds the opportunity to be grateful because these events helped you to know what you did not want in life so that you could figure out what you did and create more of that.

I grew up in a dysfunctional family that was full of emotional and physical abuse and mental disorders. From the outside, I had a very chaotic life, but from the inside, I held a future that was full of love, security, and wellbeing in the forefront of my mind at all times. My experiences helped me to get where I am today because they provided me the ability to make the changes I needed to in order to physically, emotionally, and spiritually prosper. My childhood gave me the opportunity to experience instability so that I would be able to teach people how to create the opposite. My family helped me to expand through opposition, so others could too, and I am very grateful for that.

EXERCISE:

Take a moment to reflect on your own background. Recognize that everyone in your past was doing the best they could at the time to raise you. They literally didn't know any better. If you start to implement any of the meditations in this book, you will stop interlocking with people in your life who take your energy. The meditations create a shield to protect you and give you your original power back. Anyone who was a tyrant in your life provided a fast track to make you stronger. Congratulations, you grew exponentially because the odds were against you. Next time you want to complain about your mother, father, brother, sister, boss, or friend, thank them instead. Appreciate deeply all the lessons you learned. In fact, start to bless and thank all the people that you feel hurt you in some way. Also hope that your child can do the same thing regarding your faults in the future.

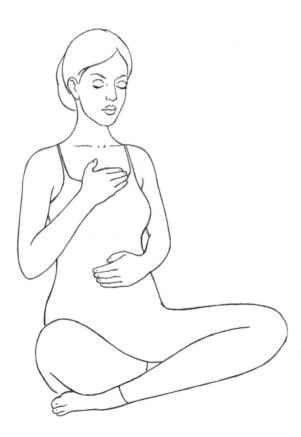

36. CULTIVATING A CREATIVE ATTITUDE

"Someone who takes the time to understand their relationship with Source, who actively seeks alignment with their Broader Perspective, who deliberately seeks and finds alignment with who-they-really-are, is more charismatic, more attractive, more effective, and more powerful than a group of millions who have not achieved that alignment."

–ABRAHAM

We are in desperate need of a different type of human being on this planet, one who is connected to their Source and brimming with unique insights. Life pours through the creative individual igniting in them a passion to serve and a commitment to make new and rapid changes on the planet. One could argue that God runs through the creative person. These individuals have a high self-confidence and self-mastery and put a great deal of unique effort into their achievements. To become a fulfilled human being who lives a no-limit life, we must cultivate creativity in ourselves. The more creative you are as a parent, the more creative your child can be. Creative individuals have a unique set of characteristics that set them apart from the masses. Here are the basic attributes of what it takes to be creative, taken from Dr. Wayne Dyer's book *What Do You Really Want for Your Children?*, a potent resource for raising a conscious child.

LIVE IN THE PRESENT MOMENT

Creative people become completely absorbed in their project and ultimately in the present moment. They don't look around to see what anyone else is doing or compare themselves to others. They live and work with intensity, lost in space and time, and have a sense of courage to create masterpieces. For them, time stands still and becomes heightened consciousness. Moments are ongoing and provide a whole and everlasting presence of flow to come through. Individuals who manifest in this way do not use the past as a reference for what they are doing now, because what they are doing now has never been done. They also don't prepare for the future because they are completely involved in the study and discovery of their creation. This is why it is important to not interrupt children when they are learning. This type of compete absorption in a project helps to cast out fears of doubts or failure.

BECOME INNOCENT LIKE A CHILD

Being open to new experiences and willing to enter unknown territory is vital to creativity. Creative people know their product will stand strong against anything that has been produced before. You must have an open perspective on life to do this and be willing to go where others have not. Being completely innocent is an attribute of the creative individual as it allows for new ideas to flow through into manifestation. The mind that does not know is ready to discover because everything is fresh and joyful. There are no names or words to describe things, because everything is new. This state of Being has been called the beginner's mind. Creative people don't look to the outside world's belief systems or dogmas for support. This is one reason not to force your children to do or believe what you do. You don't need to force religion on your children; if it is for them, they will always go toward it. If it is not, they will always rebel against it.

BECOME MORE AWARE OF YOURSELF THAN OF OTHERS

Creative individuals are fiercely independent and will not allow another to think for them. If you are interested in having the freedom to make your own decisions, you are on the right path. Children naturally want this type of expression. It is our control that limits them. To enhance creativity, you must stop looking to others for approval and focus solely on allowing Source to flow through you in a unique way. The needs of the creative are met intrinsically as they don't look to outside resources or people for happiness. When you become less aware of others, and more aware of yourself, you are on the road to creativity. Maybe you spend thirty less minutes in the mirror daily because the meditations in this book are working. That is a very positive change. A huge percentage of our energy is lost obsessing over what others are doing or thinking. When we do this, we lose a strong self-concept. If we took our power back, this energy could be put forth in new direction.

LOSE YOUR FEAR AND MOVE WITH COURAGE

Creative people have less fears, anxieties, and neurotic tendencies. They do not fear their own inherent greatness and embody their strong attributes more than the average person. If you want to become more creative, don't put limits on yourself. Things do not have to be a particular way for the creative individual; rather than being straight and narrow, they work concentrically. Think differently and let your children do this too. If there is an octopus under their bed, don't deny it; run over and take a look. Creative people are courageous with their belief systems and endeavors and almost stubborn in completing them. Their persistence in projects will exhaust all those around them, but this quality is vital to make an impact. Many great ideas are lost because people lack the inner motivation to complete tasks.

TRUST AND LETTING THINGS HAPPEN

When you are in a state of allowing and receptivity, a flow of energy will run through you to create new and adventurous projects. This type of allowing goes with the moment and does not resist the event at hand. When you try to change the moment in your mind to be different than the way it is, you are resisting and blocking the flow of energy that is consistently provided by the universe. Creative people tend to be more positive and give up criticism of themselves and others. They choose thoughts that make them feel better in all situations no matter how bad others may think it is. Doubting, choosing, correcting, and judging all take up a significant amount of internal energy. When you can go with the flow of life, you will increase your positivity and self-confidence and cultivate a unique type of power.

BE UNIQUE AND SPONTANEOUS

Being unique requires confidence, trust, and integrity. Creativity means being unique against the crowd and attacking a problem at hand from your own perspective. It is bringing something completely new into this realm. The opposite of creativity is dullness or conformity, which is a form of doing things the way we were taught. We want to teach our children to think outside the box, to even move the box to an entirely different level of awareness. Creative people become fully engaged in the project, and with no other purpose in mind are able to flow at full capacity.

EXERCISE:

Simple Ways to Enhance Creativity in Young Children

On the road to becoming a conscious parent, you must begin to move neutrally through the war zone—trying not to make the child the enemy—and accept the resistances that come up inside. Toddlers live within their own world, similar to the Little Prince, on a planet all to themselves. They are angels and then devils and are totally disorderly and completely unpredictable. In their world, they can fly, which is amazing but scary. Toddlers are creative and spectacular, and they live moment to moment. They are open to creativity at this stage, and it is our job to maintain this growth and not put limits on their imaginations.

In order to foster creativity, we need to work on ourselves first. This can be done simply through daily writing, photography, poems, books, or walks in nature. Find what you love and immerse yourself in it so you don't clock your energy. Living a creative life will then transfer to our children. Getting creative can help us to maneuver through the challenging parental moments. The more time we put into our own creativity, the more we can become creative with them—not only in the way that we respond to their unmet needs but also in the activities that we do together that help to nourish their soul. We can help to foster this aspect in our children by creating a home environment that enhances growth. Here are a few things you can implement into your home:

1. If you have small children, make sure they have a table that fits them. Place white paper out (even taped down to the table). Ensure the children have crayons or washable markers available for art. Don't be afraid to get messy.

2. Create a place in your house that has art supplies that are easy to pull out. Let them choose their activity and set up.

3. When you are with your children, or creating art, focus on playing and

not on the end product. Be present in each moment, and don't control their creations.

4. Allow them to be different—allow them to be themselves. This may help you confront your own fears about not fitting in the group.

5. Make sure your children know that creativity comes through us—not completely from us. Show them through example that they can tap into this type of energy anytime.

6. Allow unstructured play, especially outside. This type of play time allows for rest, grounding, and space.

7. Travel with them. Don't be afraid to show them new places textures, colors, sensations, sounds, or animals.

8. Read them stories made up of fantasies, imagination, myths, make-believe, or fairy tales. Make these stories come to life. Talk to the flowers and birds. Catch the imaginary beings.

9. Do not deny their imagination. Help them to expand it by letting them know that what they experience is real. Teach them about fairies, hobbits, angels, cloud castles, mysteries, and spirit. Saturate them with the unreal and improbable.

37. AN ADVANCED EDUCATION

*"Young people have joined you in your behaviors. If they are violent it is because
you are violent. If they are materialistic, it is because you are materialistic. If
they are acting crazy, it is because you are acting crazy. If they are using sex
manipulatively, irresponsibly, shamefully, it is because they see you doing the
same. The only difference between young people and older people is that young
people do what they do out in the open."*

–NEALE DONALD WALSCH, CONVERSATIONS WITH GOD

Our current education system is built upon creating memories rather than
abilities. When we do this, we teach our children knowledge without wisdom.
They learn history, facts, and figures but are not taught from an early age how
to critically analyze or problem-solve. Rather than teaching subjects, the school
system should teach concepts such as honesty, kindness, and dignity. Once these
basic personality traits are set, which are based on love, belonging, and esteem,
it would be easier and more natural to approach academic subjects. Individuals
in our society are full of facts, but they have no idea how to apply what they have
learned and create changes in the world. We keep repeating the past because we
were never encouraged to question it. When knowledge is applied, it becomes
wisdom, but when it is not, it becomes ignorance. What if children were taught

how to be aware, responsible, and honest before they learned math or English? What if they knew how to critically analyze history rather than memorize it? If this happened, we would likely create a society that would abandon our morals and beliefs in order to create better ones.

There are many parts of our current education system that should be altered in order to raise individuals that give back to their community. Little girls and boys are being pressured to learn how to read before leaving preschool and strive to memorize multiplication tables before they even understand how to treat themselves or others. The average school system functions on competition, testing standards, memorization, and historical perspective. If you had an experience like mine, you might remember long history lectures on ancient battles, in cramped rooms, that had nothing to do with the present moment. Imagine if we had been able to engage with group discussion on those battles rather than just memorizing facts that trended toward one side. If children studied the Holocaust and could critically analyze all the people and places involved, they would learn that every situation has more than one point of view. This would teach neutrality and ultimately compassion. When another genocide rises in their future, these leaders would have the tools and understanding on how to approach the issue so that history cannot repeat itself. Rather than telling our children what to think, we need to ask them what they think.

School systems of the future will not have syllabi, memorization of facts, repetition, or an organizational structure that makes teachers the only source of knowledge. They will become interactive environments where people advance through dynamic expression and open ideas. In the future individuals will learn because they love the subject. When this happens, we will ultimately build a society based on creativity and one that does not look at work as a necessity, but as a tool for growth and expansion. Neale Donald Walsch explained in the book *Conversations with God: An Uncommon Dialogue* that other than encouraging children to ask questions, we must teach them the concepts of honesty, responsibility, and awareness before we teach them subjects. If we based our school system off teaching fairness, equality, tolerance, love, and internal happiness, we would create a future full of leaders rather than followers.

Walsch explained that we must change our curriculum to be value-based rather than fact-based to create a world where we can solve conflict without violence, live without fear, act without self-interest, and love without condition. Education should be about learning to grow, understanding what to grow toward, reaching for neutrality, knowing desirable and undesirable, and learning what to choose and what not to choose through intuition. These are basic life skills.

As a parent, I understand this is going to be hard to find in our present world. I have done the school search for my children and understand the current system. If you want to find any of these qualities in a school, you have to pay a lot for it, which isn't feasible for most families. The change must start with us and at home and preferably be moved to an advanced school system in the future so that parents can avoid prejudice.

EXERCISE:

WHAT TO TEACH YOUR CHILDREN AS TAUGHT FROM CONVERSATIONS WITH GOD

√   Teach your children that they are spiritual beings having a human experience and that reality lies in their interior not exterior.

√   Teach them how the body, mind, and spirit function.

√   Make sure they understand that there is no separation and only unity.

√   Replace ownership with stewardship: Teach them that their toys are for everyone, and they are only responsible for taking care of them. Sharing will become easier as they grow if they consider everyone a loved one. Demonstrate that there is always enough so they don't grow with a fear of scarcity. Make sure that you don't assert "ownership" over your children.

√ The early images that they visualize should not be violent. This includes video games, cartoons, books, or even your home. You have to be observant of what you allow in their environment from a young age because children remember everything that they see and experience. Providing children with images of violence and rage will only teach them that this is permissible in society.

√ Children should not be rewarded based on school or sport performance but on their values.

√ Teach them that toxins such as smoking, drugs, and alcohol are harmful.

√ Children need to be taught that sex is not shameful nor are their bodies. You need to be able to express love appropriately and openly in front of them. Do not place guilt around their bowel movements, shield your own body from them, or tell them to never touch themselves. This sends them the message that pleasure and bodies are bad, which can lower their self- esteem and cause embarrassment. As the child grows older, you have to determine what feels appropriate in regards to being naked.

√ Bring out what is natural in the child such as joy, art, fairy tales, dance, expression, and music. Constantly engage them in creativity.

√ Children should learn to celebrate themselves and others. On your child's birthday have them give presents or a treat to their classmates, friends, or family rather than only receive.

√ Teach them to take into account both science and spirituality. Not everything can be proven, and some things must come from the art of knowing.

√   If their teacher puts them down, evaluate the situation, but always elevate your child. Do not let anyone talk unkindly about them.

√   Children should understand the power of their mind and that they are creative consciousness. They must understand that their thoughts and feelings are as important for the world as their actions. Just as every action has an effect so does every feeling. In this way, they will understand that when they accomplish something it is not just for their benefit but for the world.

√   Teach them visibility and transparency by being honest and true to your word. Don't lie to your children. Teach them to tell the truth and to not hold in what they are thinking or feeling but to find a way to communicate it effectively.

√   Make sure they do what they say they are going to do. Don't say one thing to them and then do another.

√   Teach your children stories based on awareness, responsibility, honesty, giving, and love. They can draw pictures about it and, as they get older, write about how each of these concepts could be carried out. Stories could be based on believing in themselves, miracles, angels, honoring others, sharing, and getting along.

√   Children should be able to critically analyze and problem solve. There is a negative and positive to every event. We cannot let children accept anything at face value, and we must teach them that there is more than one point of view on everything.

√   Children must recognize that they are connected to the whole of life. Understanding this basic concept helps people to take responsibility for everything that occurs personally or to others as a whole. One person's gain is another person's loss.

√   When it comes to work, children must also learn devotion. Work done
     for the sake of success will be the least successful, and learning done
     without devotion does not lead to progress. Only the love of work will
     lead to progress.

√   Always ask: What do you think? What do you think? What do you
     think?

√   Teach them love is all there is. Speak of a love that is unconditional.

EXERCISE:

JUPITER FINGER CHAKRA MEDITATION AS TAUGHT BY YOGI BHAJAN

*"This meditation was originally taught by Yogi Bhajan as a "children's
meditation," but can also be practiced by adolescents and adults. Anyone with
past trauma will benefit from this practice. Even someone without past trauma
can improve the balance of their personality by its use. This meditation helps to
balance the chakras and meridians in the body. It is an excellent meditation to
practice with your children. It will evoke many feelings that have stuck with you
since you were a child. It will help adults get rid of the "childhood syndrome,"
a condition where you cling to something that is already finished – a syndrome
which can easily ruin and limit your life."*

–KUNDALINI RESEARCH INSTITUTE

Please note that this meditation is not for beginners and should be taken very
seriously as it brings up a lot of old memories. If you choose to do this, start slow
and then increase your time.

Mudra: Sit straight with your eyes closed. Place your left hand flat against your chest at the heart center. Use the index (Jupiter) finger of the right hand (Keep the other fingers closed in a relaxed fist with the thumb over the other fingers.) to touch in sequence the following points:

1. The middle of the lower lip. (Chant Saa.)

2. The tip (end) of the nose. (Chant Taa.)

3. The outer edge/corner of the eye socket. (Chant Naa.)

4. A point about three-quarters of an inch above the indent of the nose, just below the forehead. (Chant Maa.)

Mantra: Chant the mantra "Saa-Taa-Naa-Maa" out loud in sequence with the touching of the points.

Since there are two eyes and thus two outer edges of the eye socket, you alternate sides each time as you go through the sequence. Start by touching the right side first. Each round of touching the points and chanting the mantra through takes about four to five seconds.

Time: Eleven to thirty-three minutes. Younger people may practice for eleven minutes or less.

End: Inhale, hold the breath, and feel your inner child by self-hypnosis. Exhale. Inhale a second time, and picture yourself as a child in your heart, where your left hand is. Concentrate. Exhale. Inhale and repeat the picture of yourself, and bless that child and yourself.

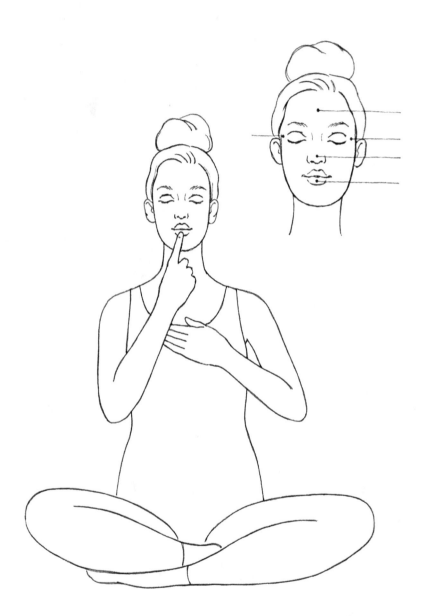

38. SPIRITUAL METAPHYSICS

"Most people don't know how deeply their own consciousness is connected to the collected fate of the planet – or how they can use a powerful, scientifically tested technology of consciousness to help create world peace on Earth virtually overnight."

–NEALE DONALD WALSCH

There is a power so profound within you, yet you do not know how to use it, nor do you even know that it exists. You are already a fully awake human; you just do not know it. This book is here to remind you of the things you have forgotten so that you can remember who you are, why you came here, and the best ways to raise the frequency of your family. What if I told you that you could heal yourself, create the world that you want, or even contribute to world peace? Do you know that you can do all of this without taking any actions? Illuminating our minds, projecting specific thoughts, and monitoring our words should be our priority. This should be some of the first things taught to children. You create what you think about, and your word is your power. This is basic spiritual technology. Imagine a future where children grow to be adults who know how to project positive thoughts, feelings, and words to create a better world. There are many examples of how the mind has healed people and communities around the world, yet we still fall short on applying this awareness to our everyday lives.

POWER OF CREATION

The first person to document how thoughts, feelings, and behavior can affect our environment was Emile Coue in in the early 1900s. Coue found that continued repetition of positive mantras and applied positive imagination could effectively heal his patients. He demonstrated through documented case studies that any idea occupying the mind turned into reality. Coue proved that positive mantras repeated out loud healed illnesses but only when the idea was consciously accepted. If the person held judgments that the thought would not come true, he could use his positive imagination to override his willpower and heal himself. Many other people have shown this throughout history, and the technology goes back to the time of Jesus and Mary.

Esther Hicks, who has been mentioned throughout this book, is a more recent teacher who has demonstrated how we can project our positive feeling and imagination to create the future we want in the present moment. Her work was so profound and far-reaching that a famous movie and book called The Secret was created based on her explanation of this reality. The movie made it clear that if you really wanted a diamond necklace and you felt with all your heart that you already had it, a necklace would magically appear. This is true; a necklace will appear if you feel and believe it. Small personal creations are not going to change the dynamics of this planet though, and we need to utilize this spiritual technology to create large positive changes.

What you put your mind on you magnify. When we do this as a group, we can create war or peace. There is vast amount of evidence that when people come together with a focused positive intention there is a drastic decrease in warfare and terror on the planet. The unified field of Consciousness is an ocean of intelligence. What you speak out, the Universe will send in. This is your creative power. When the individual mind aligns with this field, it is only natural that every thought or action would be supported. This is law. More than fifty demonstrated projects and twenty-three published studies in leading peer-reviewed journals have demonstrated that when large peace-creating meditative groups come together for a period of time there is a decrease in ethnic, political, and religious tensions. In turn, terrorism, violence, and war will decrease. This group-consciousness-based approach to peace has been proven effective on local, state, national and international levels, and each time there has been significant drops in negative social trends. You can read more on this through the Permanent Peace Organization. It starts with you. What you teach your children could make or break our future. Our personal consciousness affects the planet, and we can no longer live in this dream of separation.

THE EFFECTS OF REPEATING NEGATIVE THOUGHTS

Neale Donald Walsch explained in the book *Conversations with God Book 4* that the fastest way to wake up from this slumber is to help another person wake up. This becomes difficult when we are stuck in a negative mindset and literally do not have the motivation or power to help ourselves. When we are negative or depressed, and believe the world is out to get us, it takes a significant amount of energy to lift us out of this loop. It is hard to elevate ourselves because we keep letting everybody know how bad it is. We yearn to feel our own anger and pain through conversations with others to prove to ourselves that we have the right to feel this way. I know you have a friend who keeps picking the wrong men. We all do. She likes to complain about them, let you know how hard it is, and tell you specifics about all the awful things they do. You, in turn, agree with the way she feels, thus proving her point and creating relief, so the loop goes on. Press repeat.

Individuals are always trying to have a bigger experience of what they are feeling inside whether it is love or hate. If someone feels abandoned or angry, like your friend above, they will look to re-live and relieve that pressure through communication with you. We are all basically repeating the same story and belief systems with new actors and places throughout our lives. Good news is we are just one thought away from making massive leaps in our Consciousness. In order to change this pattern within yourself, first you need to decide what you want to have a bigger experience of in life. When you are ready to have a bigger experience of pleasure, joy, abundance, or freedom, reflect this out through your thoughts, actions, and words. Each person offers the opportunity to reflect this back to you because you attract what you are. This is a fundamental principle that all children should learn.

YOUR SUBCONSCIOUS MIND AFFECTS YOUR THOUGHTS

Speaking negatively does not hurt the person you are talking to; ii only hurts you. It will destroy your energy field. Children should learn from a young age the importance of respecting others through their words and actions. When we speak about traumatic events that happened ten years ago, we are locked in a time distortion and broadcasting to the Universe to bring more of the same. By default, the mind goes negative first because it is natural for human beings to want to protect themselves from danger. This is important for crossing the street or meeting strangers. It becomes tricky when we let it rule us. Imagine you meet someone from your past who hurt you. The negative mind will run through all the reasons this person is bad even though it may not be true in the present moment. It loves data to prove its point. It takes a significant amount of energy to redirect the negative mind to a positive or neutral place because our subconscious is full of garbage that has not been cleaned out through meditation. Yogi Bhajan taught that when the subconscious mind starts getting full, it will unload into the unconscious. This then unloads to the conscious, which is your waking world. When this happens, you suffer nightmares daily. The subconscious mind holds all your memories, events, patterns, and beliefs that you may not even be aware exist. When these are not released, they will overflow to other parts of our life creating neurosis, obsessions, depression, or negativity. When you are so full and heavy, you can't help but repeat the same mistakes, patterns, or language throughout your life.

HOW TO CHANGE YOUR THOUGHTS

Your thoughts are all there is in life. They have created your entire world. Expression is a thought, and every thought is backed up with feelings, emotions, and desires. What we communicate to other people has a deeper effect on us than anybody else. Teach your children this. If you need to release your negative stories and have the urge to tell someone, go speak to a tree. The tree will likely listen better. If you are polluting someone when you speak, you are only polluting yourself. The words you say can heal or cause disease. Negative words literally negate you. If your words are full of grace and love and backed with positive feelings, you will never get in trouble and will have a prosperous and abundant life.

Meditation and mantra is the fastest and easiest way to raise your vibration and release your subconscious mind. It will create enough internal energy to switch you from the negative mind to a more positive or neutral place of creation. I have already demonstrated how meditation can help to deactivate your issues throughout the book, but you must also understand that mantra is a coded sound within the larger sound system of infinity. It is a projection that goes to the universe and brings back a message. Teach your children to catch these messages through the example of your actions.

The things that you hear affect your body, and the words that you speak affect your nervous system. Mantra creates new mental waves and neural pathways. This new vibration will make every cell of your body dance with a positive rhythm. When you say positive words, you begin to vibrate differently. This will change the people, places, and events you attract in your life. You literally begin to upgrade yourself to a new reality. Jesus tried to teach this. Sages throughout history have attempted to show us. Emile Coue even proved this in 1900s, but nobody had the energy or motivation to follow through. Kundalini mantras will provide you with that energy, and they are very easy to incorporate into your life. You can just turn them on in your house or car, and you will feel an immediate switch in the environment because your cells will begin to dance with a new vibration. You may even like the music and begin to sing along, and so will your children. Your children crave this kind of joy, and they already know the words, because it is coded in them. Mantra will change your mental projection because it cuts through the repeated negative thoughts and projects grace to infinity. Welcome to your new life.

EXERCISE:

Further Points to Understand and Teach Your Children

- √   Your internal and external dialogue affects your experience, and this metaphysical understanding should be the first thing taught to children.

- √   When you are in control of your mood and senses, you will automatically become more intuitive. Intuition requires a calm mind.

- √   Don't talk to let it out. If you need to be emotional, go stand in nature. The trees will listen to you better than a human being will.

- √   Therapists help to release the initial understanding that you have a problem. If you keep going back to tell them about the same problem, you are only creating it. You are also losing your money.

- √   When you speak, aim to a have a positive feeling behind your words. If you want to speak from the heart, say it until something happens within you. If you believe what you are saying, something shifts in you, and then it will shift in the other person. When something comes out of you, it needs to come from a genuine place so that nature can support your effort. Try this with your children, and see how they respond.

√ Teach your children that everything is energy in vibration. Always pay attention to what you say, think, and do to create a positive vibration.

√ Make a list of all the patterns you repeat in your life with variations of the actors and scenes. Your issues will arise again. Instead of reacting the same way, plan how you will respond. Are you going to be calm, understanding, accepting, and peaceful the next time the event occurs?

√ Don't entertain the negative thoughts in your mind. When a negative thought arises, deliberately change your mind about it. Always ask if the thought is true. One hundred percent of the time it is not because there is always an opposite.

√ Kundalini Yoga, Meditation, and Mantra provide you with energy to see what is true and what is not true in you. Kundalini Yoga is just one way, but it is not the only way. There are many roads to awakening. When you sit with yourself in meditation, you can find out where your problems lie and the patterns you repeat.

39. QUALITIES IN AN AWAKENED HUMAN

"Don't ask what the world needs. Ask what makes you come alive, and go do it. Because what the world needs is people who have come alive."

–HOWARD THURMAN

The process of awakening to yourself and a deeper connection to the world feels like moving back veils while walking down a long dark hall. Similar to peeling an onion, you must work to get to the finer layers. When you walk through this tunnel, you know there is light at the end, but you cannot always see your way. Trusting that you are heading down a road that will eventually provide a heightened experience of being more present on earth will help to accelerate your growth. My awakening arrived like a series of atomic bombs that blinded me over many years. The process was painful, isolating, and confusing. Now the light pours in. I am able to see what I came here to do. I no longer feel separation and want more than ever to serve you, because you are ultimately me.

Before this, I was stuck in repetitive patterns in relationships, career, and life. When I reflect on the challenges, I can see clearly now that they helped to accelerate my progress. I did not mature in a sequential order but rather in a series of exponential growth periods. Everyone's awakening process varies. Different characters play in each of our stories. The end goal is the same: to know God and to feel yourself as the Beloved on this earth. On the sacred path to awakening, you will shed density to become lighter, experience wholeness, and feel a love so profound it will open your heart in ways you could not dream of before.

TAKE ON THE CHALLENGES

Challenges force you to learn and approach the world in an alternative way. Creating new life through motherhood provides one of the greatest opportunities to dive in and find your own truth. My journey to awakening started a few years before I became a mother and intensified with each child. It is often the baby's energy that sparks an interest in spirituality for the woman. The soul you carry within you and take care of is directly connected to Spirit and can help you mature at a greater pace. Children are alive and awake, and it is our job to let them remain that way. I will expand further on important values and concepts we should teach our children when it comes to the larger essence we call God, Spirit, or the Universe. You must foster this connection for your children in the early years so that they gain a deep trust for themselves and find their purpose here on earth. If your child sees that you are committed to growth, they will follow. Awakened humans hold specific qualities that you can cultivate in yourself and your family. As you can see by now, this book is just as much about your awakening as it is your child's.

DEVOTION TO THE PATH

To understand truth and knowledge, you must commit to the path of growth and not become impatient with how long the process takes. Rudolf Steiner explained in his book *How to Know Higher Worlds* that devotion is the fundamental attitude for growth of the soul. Devotion is a choice to commit to increasing wisdom, love, and higher values in your life for the sake of yourself and all others. Commitment means leaning into infinity. This decision will bring you trust in something much larger than yourself and immense expansion. Steiner said, "If we do not develop within ourselves this deeply rooted feeling that there is something higher than ourselves, we shall never find the strength to evolve to something higher." Devoting yourself to awakening is a process that starts out with small daily changes. These modifications feel so good that eventually every moment can become a meditation, act of splendor, or reason for joy. These feelings can only be tapped into now, because in time and space, now is all there is. When you approach life with devotion, you will begin to have appreciation and awe for every person, place, and encounter. You can teach your children this by slowing down and taking the time to notice the beauty in these experiences. The more devoted you are to the path of awakening, the higher you can climb on the mountain of knowledge. Climbing to the top also brings many peak experiences or a sudden understanding of the secrets of the universe.

PEAK EXPERIENCES

Peak experiences are filled with emotions and epiphanies, which bring feelings of expansion, oceanic bliss, and loss of self. Abraham Maslow explained that individuals who are fulfilled or self-actualized have more of these mystical peak experiences than the average person. These moments in time play out as anything that comes close to an experience of perfection such as looking at the ocean, natural childbirth, or falling in love. Mystics have had these experiences throughout time and so can you. They happen when you connect to a lager force and vibrate the body at a higher speed. They also help to drop personal neurotic tendencies because individuals become connected and feel whole again. These moments of illumination provide increased awareness, intrinsic reward, and massive internal changes. Both peak experiences and devotion can be cultivated by taking your children to holy places on earth, walking in nature, listening to music, or deep venerated love toward another. You must teach your children to be a seeker of these higher experiences, which provide an opportunity for transformation and reverence.

Every time we seek higher consciousness, we are getting closer to higher knowledge. Powers will remain dormant until you are a devoted student to the path of self-discovery. You can teach your children to remain connected to their inner and outer life by demonstrating that you stop to breathe, meditate, or pray. Show them that the natural expressions of life bring awe and wonder by pausing to reflect. If they see you taking the time for appreciation or devotion, they will too. As you create an intimate relationship with the self, you will also find that the phenomena of the outer world has a deeper meaning and splendor. Your inner world will unlock the eternal language of the cosmic spirit. Imagine what earth would be like if the next generation had the ability to understand this language early on.

INTUITION

The Universe is constantly speaking, but very few know how to listen. Most of us were never taught all the ways that God speaks to us. You can change that pattern now by tuning into this universal language and teaching your children how to connect to the signs and symbols or intuitive knowing. Intuition is a fast insight or immediate understanding and is a common way for spirit to speak to us. It often comes in the form of a feeling, inner voice, or picture. We must teach our children that they have an inner guidance system, which can help them navigate through the rough patches of life. God speaks in unlimited ways. Insight may come from the lyrics of music, symbols, books, nature, dreams, or people. When we listen to God, we have to step back and feel what is going on in our body. These sensations provide clues as to whether we are on the right track. Do not brush off these experiences as coincidences. This sign language should not be considered an accident but a common occurrence. Synchronicities are tactics that the Universe uses to get our attention and lead us in the right direction. Children should learn to expect miracles.

COMMUNICATION WITH GOD

One way to cultivate this inner guidance system within your children is to teach them from a young age that they can always and readily communicate with the Universe. Neale Donald Walsch explained in the book *Conversations with God for Parents* that in order to do this, parents must first have some clarity about who they are and what their belief systems about God, life, and death are. If you have established yourself deeply in your own soul, then you will have a greater understanding that we are all one, and death is a continuation of life. When the mind, body, and soul are in balance, it becomes easier to project this wholeness and teach from a place of authenticity. Children will be able to tell if you are coming from a place of truth when you are teaching them, so it is important to practice what you preach.

Walsch explained that when talking about Spirit, you can make God into a person rather than a larger essence so that the subject becomes more tangible to understand. Speak directly to God out loud while cooking or doing household chores. Make it a normal occurrence to tell Spirit how thankful you are. Speak about Spirit openly so that your children know holding this conversation is normal and expected. Teach your children to use their imagination in a way that they know that God is on their side. If they want something, let them know that they can use their will, positive imagination, feelings, and projection to communicate their needs. Explain that the Universe will give them what is best for them and often it is not what they think they want but what they need. Use stories to discuss the high qualities of awakened individuals such as love, compassion, or truth. Stories from great historical figures can be used as an example, and role-playing can be implemented.

All people have a desire to be at one with a greater force. You should pull out these innate qualities over time rather than try to force the connection in your child. Devotion and cultivation of higher spiritual qualities will help your child excel in life. If we teach children these characteristics at a young age, they will be on a fast track to living the life of their dreams.

EXERCISE:

Here Are Some Specific Practices That You Can Do to Create a Deeper Communication with the Universe. These Exercises Can Be Taught to Children Over Time and Especially as They Grow.

1. Look at a flower or plant as intently as possible, and let the feelings and thoughts that are provoked take possession of you. Focus on objects that blossom and flourish and those that decay and die. Pay attention to the spaces in between. Do this exercise continually over a long period of time, and you will find that new thoughts and feelings will eventually arise. When you surrender to these thoughts and feelings, while becoming one with what you are looking at, you are essentially connecting to the world of the soul or astral plane. This act helps to enhance clairvoyance and increase intuition, or the power to see objects and events that cannot be perceived by the senses. It will also help you to understand that feelings and thoughts create reality in the physical realm. Over time, with practice, you will see significant spiritual results that can be transferred to all objects in your sight.

2. Transfer this exercise to all inanimate objects. Start looking at stones, and notice the feelings and thoughts that arise. At first these feelings and thoughts only last as long as you stare, but over time, this connection will remain living in your soul. Move up from observing the plants, stones, animals, and then the spiritual world. What was

formerly invisible becomes visible. You will gain spiritual insight into the soul of others and appreciate the spiritual essence in everything.

3. Concentrate on the sounds around you and the fact that they communicate pleasure or pain. Don't pay attention to the emotion behind the sound; just listen intently. You will begin to intermingle with the being and its sound current. When you listen to inanimate objects, nature, or people fully, you will become aware of a unified field that speaks the language of the soul. This is especially important when listening to people speak. Become silent and drop all judgments. When you practice listening without criticism, you can blend yourself with another and develop a new sense of hearing. When you are unmoved by the sound or opinions in the world, the universe will recognize itself in you. Through this inner stillness and silence, higher sources and beings will begin to communicate with you. This is called clairaudience, or hearing outside the range of normal perception.

40. HEAL YOURSELF,
HEAL THE WORLD

"If you could get rid of yourself just once, the secret of secrets would open to you. The face of the unknown, hidden beyond the universe would appear on the mirror of your perception."

–RUMI

A Letter to All Mothers,

I remember the day it happened. I was helping a beautiful young woman pack her bags while she held her new baby proudly in her arms after breastfeeding. We laughed as I dressed her seven-pound angel. It crossed my mind that we would be good friends, if I wasn't her nurse, if we weren't in this cold hospital room, and if she wasn't about to be discharged. Her husband left to get the car, and her guard dropped. The tears exploded as she fell to the bed. My instinct was to fall with her, let down any professional guard, and meet her at the heart level. I held her while she sobbed. I felt an unhealed pain in her so profound that I cried too. You see, this woman had been in the hospital for over twelve days after complications from her birth. She lost over six liters of blood, was sent to the intensive care unit, battled infections and the possibility of death, and was separated from her new child the entire time. The doctors had left a needle in her. One intervention cascaded into another, and she lost her power. She was also being sent home with no resources to help her understand what had happened.

This woman was a warrior, and her birth story proved it. It was also a secret that she would carry throughout life because she felt no one else would under-stand. I asked if she had any support at home, someone to listen. She didn't want to speak of it again publicly and explained that she would never have another child. Like every mother out there, she wanted her birth to be valued. I know she buried her pain in hopes that she would never have to face it again. We all know that she will though.

I met this patient years ago, but she represents millions of people all over the earth who need to heal their stories. If one person hurts, we all do. After meeting her, I knew we had to do things differently. I knew there was a better way, and I became determined to teach women how to birth a new consciousness into this world. This patient showed me how it should not be done so that I could find out how it should be done. You have read my findings, which I was guided to by a higher source so that everyone could benefit and alter their approach to motherhood.

Since that encounter, I have worked with many women who have had similar experiences and carry a tremendous amount of burden. Their stories are different, but the pain is the same. Whether it is multiple miscarriages, lost children, rape, sexual abuse, or painful relationships, women carry a great amount of their past in their womb. Until everyone of these women are healed, and the matrix is con-nected, there will always be more work to do. When we heal ourselves, we are also healing Mother Earth. Life is an ongoing process of choosing between safety, out of fear, and growth. I hope you have learned through this book the importance of always choosing growth. If you do this, and teach your children this too, life will become vivid and alive. Your real self will emerge. A highly functioning human being transcends their wounds, story, and culture. This work is more important than we consciously understand because most of us don't have a grasp on the fact that there is no separation. When one woman rises, she takes an army with her.

The same patterns will arise in your life until you face them. We must heal individually and as a collective culture. Our challenges provide an opportunity to wake up and our biggest adversities give us a mirror to go deeper into our triggers. This woman's story is important because it represents how unconsciously we tend to approach the most sacred act on this planet and the personal consequences it can have on a family. I wrote this book to help you see that there is always an alternative, and there are many values to incorporate in your life on the road to conscious parenting. If you take even one of these sections seriously and apply it to your life, you are making a tremendous effort to change and standing out from the crowd. When you start to confront yourself as you would a stranger, you can see your own patterns of self-sabotage. As you start to go inward, you will cultivate a great strength, and what used to anger or annoy you will no longer hold that power. Whether or not you have experienced trauma, there is something in you that needs to be peeled back and approached with care so that you can become a more conscious mother. Until you understand yourself and your own belief systems, how could you possibly teach your children from a place of honesty or knowing? Children will always look to you for guidance and certainty. Know yourself: your reactions, patterns, and belief systems matter. When you do, you will also know how much power you hold as leader for your family.

This book provides you with steps to follow on your road to motherhood so that you can become a conscious example and raise fulfilled human beings. All people who persevere on the road to awakening will develop new skills. A new light will likely envelop you or your child and reveal an organ of sight, which provides access to the presence of various dimensions of existence that you were not aware even existed. Creating and caring for children is a spiritual journey that offers women the opportunity to explore their strengths and weaknesses. A journey so sacred it creates a glimpse into our deepest selves. There are a variety of ways to excavate your past to create a new reality in the present. We have gone through many examples and approaches on how to change your life throughout this text. If you haven't taken the opportunity to complete these exercises, or experience these meditations, I encourage you to go back at any time and explore. This book is meant to shape your life for a long period of time. If it speaks to your heart, share your new power and insights so that other women who are ready to heal and awaken can join you. There is an army of individuals who are getting prepared to do things differently in this world, and they need your help. You don't have to claim to be leader; you just have to show them that you went first so that they can follow. The fastest way to accelerate your own growth is to teach someone else. That is how a master is born.

When you win the inner world, you win the outer world. Both places are confinement, but you must conquer them. The only way to be successful in the outer world is to conquer your inner world first. Once this happens, you will find that you no longer have to do anything to move forward; you just have to be a little more open to receiving abundance. Crystalize yourself. This comes with an honest and open craving to awaken to who you truly are in any given moment, which is always growing and expanding. When you know this, you know God.

Don't get depressed if you make a mistake or feel that you are not growing fast enough as a person or a parent. Give yourself some credit for how far you have come. Make sure your children always know how much you love them, that you are doing your best in the moment, and that you are attempting to become a better version of yourself. If you weren't, you would not be sitting here reading this book. When you heal, or face your life challenges with vigor, you will also heal the generations that are before and after you. Remember who you are. Remember that you are a woman and a creator. You hold infinity in your womb and the power to change this planet. One mother at a time, we will birth a new reality. This is a revolution, and you are the change makers.

IMAGINE A WOMAN

Imagine a woman who believes it is right and good she is a woman. A woman who honors her experience and tells her stories. Who refuses to carry the sins of others within her body and life.

Imagine a woman who trusts and respects herself. A woman who listens to her needs. Who meets them with tenderness and grace.

Imagine a woman who has acknowledged the past's influence on the present. A woman who has walked through her past. Who has healed into the present.

Imagine a woman who authors her own life. A woman who exerts, initiates, and moves on her own behalf. Who refuses to surrender except to her truest self and wisest voice.

Imagine a woman who names her own gods. A woman who imagines the Divine in her image and likeness. Who designs a personal spirituality to inform her daily life.

Imagine a woman in love with her own body. A woman who believes her body is enough just as it is. Who celebrates her body's rhythms and cycles as an exquisite resource.

Imagine a woman who honors the body of the Goddess in her changing body. A woman who celebrates the accumulation of her years and her wisdom. Who refuses to use her precious life energy disguising the changes in her body and life.

Imagine a woman who values the woman in her life. A woman who sits in circles of women. Who is reminded of the truth about herself when she forgets.

Imagine yourself as this woman.

Patricia Reilly

FERTILE

Pritam's newest book is available for purchase on Amazon and through the Mystical Motherhood website.

Fertile: Prepare Your Body, Mind, and Spirit for Conception and Pregnancy to Create a Conscious Child

Fertile is a revolutionary approach to conscious motherhood. Applying visionary concepts to fertility and pregnancy, Pritam Atma shares a beautifully illustrated guide to heal your body, mind, and spirit in preparation for pregnancy and creating an enlightened child. This book opens a doorway into the unknown mysteries of creation.

This book is written for women who are struggling with fertility, want to consciously conceive, and those who are already pregnant. It is applicable to women who have no children and those who want more. The transformational process can be utilized whether you become pregnant naturally or with medical help from intrauterine insemination, in vitro fertilization or an egg donor.

Pritam introduces a new paradigm by teaching women that they are the genetic engineers of their babies during pregnancy. This modern approach to motherhood gives women their power back. Learn how to consciously create a child with thoughts and emotions based on love and harmony.

From diet and mental health—to career and relationships—*Fertile* balances every aspect of your life to increase fertility and dramatically alter your approach to pregnancy, birth, and motherhood. Explore unique ways to transform by increasing your happiness and well-being during the most critical period of your child's development.

Combining cutting-edge scientific theory with sacred spiritual revelations, this is a road map to activating your divine role as a mother. Whether this is your first child or your third, *Fertile* is designed explicitly for all women who are ready to awaken to their divinity and improve this planet by creating highly conscious children.

- Apply emerging scientific research on behavioral epigenetics to pregnancy. Learn how to improve your child's consciousness by changing your thoughts, beliefs, emotions, environment, and diet.

- Enhance your nutrition, heal generational patterns and increase your level of spirituality in preparation for conscious motherhood.

- Understand the transformative power of alchemy and learn how the elements, your level of sensory awareness,and sacred geometry help to design your child.

- Master your thoughts and increase your level of awareness by projecting an experience based on love, rather than fear, for your growing child during pregnancy.

- Improve your relationship through enhanced intimacy and heightened sexuality. Create the Holy Trinity through the activation of the divine masculine, divine feminine and holy child.

REFERENCES

SECTION 1

Bhajan, Yogi. (2017) *Andaj Kriya. Creating the Aquarian Child Course Manual.* Unpublished. Rama Institute of Applied Technology.

Bhajan, Yogi. (2017) *Gurprassad Meditation. Creating the Aquarian Child Course Manual.* Unpublished. Rama Institute of Applied Technology.

Bhajan, Yogi. (2008). *Meditation for Healing Addictions.* Healthy, Happy Holy Organization. Retrieved from https://www.3ho.org/3ho-lifestyle/health-and-healing/meditation-healing-addictions-0

Bhajan, Yogi. (2002). *Sat Kriya.* Kundalini Research Institute National Training Manual Level 1. Retrieved from *http://www.kundaliniresearchinstitute.org/newsletter/2014/Sat-Kriya.pdf*

Junger, Alejandro. (2014). *Clean Gut: The Breakthrough Plan for Eliminating the Root Cause of Disease and Revolutionizing Your Health.* (Kindle DX version). Retrieved from Amazon.

Maslow, Abraham. (1970). *Motivation and Personality.* New York City. Longman.

Northrup, Christian. (2010). *Women's Bodies, Women's Wisdom (Revised Edition): Creating Physical and Emotional Health and Healing* (Kindle DX version). Retrieved from Amazon.

Richardson, Kelly. (2017). *What Clutter is Trying to Tell You: Uncover the Message in the Mess and Reclaim Your Life.* (Kindle DX version). Retrieved from Amazon.

Roberts, J. (1972). *Seth Speaks the Eternal Validity of the Soul.* (Kindle DX version). Retrieved from Amazon.

Singh, Guru. (2017). *21st Century Prophets: The Sage Within.* ReEvolution Books.

Villoldo, A. (2015). *One Spirit Medicine: Ancient Ways to Ultimate Wellness.* (Kindle DX version). Retrieved from Amazon.

K, T., K.H., K.G., J., J.G. (2017). *Creating the Aquarian Child Course Manual.* (Unpublished Manual). Rama Institute of Applied Technology. Los Angeles, CA.

Werner-Gray, L., (2014) *Earth Diet: Your Complete Guide to Living Using Earth's Natural Ingredients.* (Kindle DX version). Retrieved from Amazon.

William, Anthony. (2016). *Medical Medium: Life-Changing Foods: Save Yourself and The Ones You Love with the Hidden Healing Powers of Fruits and Vegetables.* (Kindle DX version). Retrieved from Amazon.

William, Anthony. (2015). *Medical Medium: Secrets Behind Chronic and Mystery Illness and How to Finally Heal.* (Kindle DX version). Retrieved from Amazon.

SECTION 2

Bhajan, Yogi. (2016). *I am a Woman Affirmation Practice.* The Yogi Bhajan Library of Teachings. Retrieved from *https://www.libraryofteachings.com/kriya.xqy?q=%20sort:titleAscending&id=536d1cf8-3dfa-35b1-b3bc-4f2d68c-3f9af&name=I-am-a-Woman:-Affirmation-Practice*

Bhajan, Yogi. (2008). *Kirtan Kriya*. Kundalini Research Institute. Retrieved from http://kundaliniresearchinstitute.org/wp-content/uploads/2017/04/KirtanKriya.pdf

Gaskin, Ina May. (2011). *Birth Matters: A Midwife's Manifesta*. New York City. Seven Stories Press.

Bhajan, Yogi. (2017). ***The Divine Shield Meditation for Protection and Positivity. Healthy, Happy Holy Organization. Retrieved from*** https://www.3ho.org/divine-shield-meditation-protection-and-positivity

Bhajan, Yogi. (2018). *Meditation for Dire Depression. Creating the Aquarian Child Manual*. Unpublished. Rama Institute of Applied Technology.

Caughey, A. B., Cahill, A. G., Guise, J., Rouse, D. J., (2014). *Safe Prevention of the Primary Cesarean Delivery. Number 1.* The American College of Obstetrics and Gynecologists. Retreived from ***https://www.acog.org/Resources-And-Publications/Obstetric-Care-Consensus-Series/Safe-Prevention-of-the-Primary-Cesarean-Delivery***

Huddleston, Peggy. (1996) *Prepare for Surgery, Heal Faster: A Guide to Mind Body Techniques*. Angel River Press. MA

K, T., K.H., K.G., J., J.G. (2017). *Creating the Aquarian Child Course Manual.* (Unpublished Manual). Rama Institute of Applied Technology. Los Angeles, CA.

Walsh, Denis. (2012). *Evidence and Skills for Normal Labour and Birth a Guide for Midwives*. New York City. Routledge.

Klaus, M, M.D. and Kennell, J. (2017). Special Role of the Doula. Retrieved from *http://www.bondingandbirth.org/doulas.html*

Northrup, Christian. (2010). *Women's Bodies, Women's Wisdom (Revised Edition): Creating Physical and Emotional Health and Healing* (Kindle DX version). Retrieved from Amazon.

SECTION 3

Bhajan, Yogi. (2017). *Meditation to Release Childhood Anger.* Sourced from Meditation as Medicine. Retrieved from http://www.shaktakaur.com/meditations/release_the_past_especially_childhood_anger.htm

Bhajan, Yogi. (1976). *Meditation to Preventing Freaking Out.* Kundalini Research

Institute Crisis Kit. Retrieved from *http://kundaliniresearchinstitute.org/docs/KRI-Crisis-Kit.pdf*

Brown, Brene. (2015). *Daring Greatly: How the Courage to Be Vulnerable Transforms the Way We Live, Love, Parent, and Lead.* (Kindle DX version). Retrieved from Amazon.

Hicks, Esther. and Hicks, Jerry. (2009) *The Vortex Where the Law of Attraction Assembles All Cooperative Relationships.* (Kindle DX version). Retrieved from Amazon.

Kaur Khlasa, Tarn Taran. (2006). *Call Upon the Maha Shakti as taught by Yogi Bhajan.* Conscious Pregnancy Yoga Manual. 3HO Women. New Mexico.

Oakes and Khanolkar. (2009). *Touching Heaven Tonic and Delicious Postpartum Recipes from Ayurveda.* Sacred Window Ayruveda for Mothers and Children.

SECTION 4

Bhajan, Yogi. (2003) *I am Happy Meditation for Children. Healthy, Happy Holy Organization. Retrieved from https://www.3ho.org/3ho-lifestyle/healthy-happy-holy-lifestyle/happy/three-meditations-happiness*

Bhajan, Yogi. (2017). *Meditation for Thinking Before You Speak.* Spirit Voyage. Retrieved from http://www.spiritvoyage.com/blog/index.php/think-before-you-speak-kundalini-yoga-for-conscious-communication/

K, T., K.H., K.G., J., J.G. (2017). *Creating the Aquarian Child Course Manual.* (Unpublished Manual). Rama Institute of Applied Technology. Los Angeles, CA.

Liedloff, Jean. (2008). *The Continuum Concept: In Search of Happiness Lost (Classics in Human Development.* (Kindle DX version). Retrieved from Amazon.

Fleming P, Blair P, Mckenna J. *New knowledge, new insights, and new recommendations: Scientific controversy and media hype in unexpected infant deaths.* Arch Dis Child. 2006;91(10):799-801.

McKenna J., McDade T._Why babies should never sleep alone: a review of the co-sleeping controversy in relation to SIDS, bedsharing and breast feeding.* Rev. 2005 Jun;6(2):134-52.

University of Notre Dame. (2017). *Safe Cosleeping Guidelines. Retrieved from http://cosleeping.nd.edu/safe-co-sleeping-guidelines*

SECTION 5

Bhajan, Yogi. *Jupiter Finger Chakra Meditation.* Yogamint. Retrieved from *http://www.yogamint.com/video/jupiter-finger-chakra-meditation*

Dyer, Wayne. (2001). *What Do You Really Want for Your Children?* (Kindle DX version). Retrieved from Amazon.

Coue, E. (date unknown). *Self-Mastery Through Conscious Autosuggestion.* Retrieved from http://brainybetty.com/2007Motivation/Emile%20Coue%20-%20Self%20Mastery.pdf

Hicks, Esther. and Hicks, Jerry. (2009) *The Vortex Where the Law of Attraction Assembles All Cooperative Relationships.* (Kindle DX version). Retrieved from Amazon.

Maslow, Abraham. (1970). *Motivation and Personality.* New York City. Longman.

Pearce, J. C. (1992). *Magical Child.* New York City. Plume.

Permanent Peace. (2017). What's the Evidence? Retrieved from *http://permanent-peace.org/evidence/index.html*

Steiner, R. (1910). *How to Know Higher Wolds.* (Kindle DX version). Retrieved from Amazon.

Walsch, N. D. (1997). *Conversations with God: An Uncommon Dialogue Book 2.* (Kindle DX version). Retrieved from Amazon.

Walsch, N. D. (2016). *Conversations with God: An Uncommon Dialogue Book 4.* (Kindle DX version). Retrieved from Amazon.

Walsch, N. D., Farley, L.L., Filmore, E. (1995). *Conversations with God for Parents: Sharing the Messages with Children.* (Kindle DX version). Retrieved from Amazon.

APPRECIATION

My life has been full of opportunities of inspiration that led me to write this book. I am very grateful to my family and friends in Utah who helped to create a foundation for me to work from as I grew in life. Thank you to my teachers and fellow students I met while studying nursing in Los Angeles. I appreciate all the patients who I met along the way through my career and education that gave me personal insight into the tribulations and triumphs at birth. Thank you to Ina May Gaskin, Yogi Bhajan, and all my spiritual teachers who helped me grow exponentially in order to be prepared to embody this work. I appreciate my husband dearly for allowing me the space and stability to explore my dream to serve others in this manner. Thank you to my two children who birthed new consciousness through me. These angels helped me to understand that there are countless ways of improving. Most importantly, I thank God, the Goddess, and the Universe for guiding me on this path and directly coaching me through completing this book.

CONNECT WITH US

To find out more about all of this, visit Mystical Motherhood online. If you are interested in private sessions, group sessions, classes, or retreats please contact us. Pritam works with women all over the world helping them to heal on profound levels. See below for further information.

www.mysticalmotherhood.com

Facebook: Mystical Motherhood

Instagram: @mysticalmotherhood

Twitter: @mysticalmother1

Email: mysticalmotherhood @ gmail.com

Mystical Motherhood Podcast is on Itunes

CPSIA information can be obtained
at www.ICGtesting.com
Printed in the USA
LVHW011536280820
664254LV00008B/665